A

GW00712275

Twisted
Cross

~

J. R. Russell

~

Published in 2013 by Skycat Publications
Vaiseys Farm, Brent Eleigh, Suffolk CO10 9 PA
Email info@skycatpublications.com
www.skycatpublications.com

ISBN 978 0 9575673 0 6

Digitally printed by Book Printing UK
Remus House, Coltsfoot Drive, Woodston, Peterborough PE2 9BF
Email: info@BookPrintingUK.com
Telephone: 01733 898102   Fax: 01733 313524

© 2013 J. R. Russell

Cover designed by Kitty Best

~

Contents

~

~

List of Characters

Officers & Gentlemen
Lord Robert of St Foy
Lord Aimery, brother to Robert
Count Louis of Blois
Count Hugh of St Pol
Count Baldwin of Flanders
Boniface Marquis of Montferrat
Enrico Dandolo, Doge of Venice

Soldiers and Rogues
Kit
Bishop
Lawyer
Merchant
Poet
Deuce
Soldier
Gentleman

Byzantine Emperors
Alexius III (1195-1203)
Isaac II (1203-1204)
Alexius IV (1203-1204)
Alexius V, Mourtzouphlus (1204)
Nicolas Canabus (6 days 1204)

~

~

Introduction

THIS is a story told by a child of a great crime committed in the name of God. In this it is signal but not unique, in these days almost a commonplace.

A Christian crusade called by Pope Innocent III in 1199 to redeem the holy city of Jerusalem ended five years later in the siege and occupation of the Christian city of Constantinople, capital of the Byzantine Empire. An army of devoted men enlisted in an honourable cause was diverted to a desperate and dishonourable action ending in robbery, rape and murder, and the destruction of a culture and an empire. The great cathedral of St Sophia was desecrated and despoiled, churches and libraries were ravaged, statues, monuments and mosaics were shattered, precious relics of ancient Greece and early Christianity were stolen and scattered throughout Europe, the vast wealth of a thousand years of empire was seized and squandered, a whole population was dispersed, a whole civilisation was destroyed.

How did it happen?

Here, a child, a little Christian, is led by faith into a maze of power, of greed, of necessity, of arrogance and stupidity, where the only way out is the one most dreaded, the loss of faith itself.

~

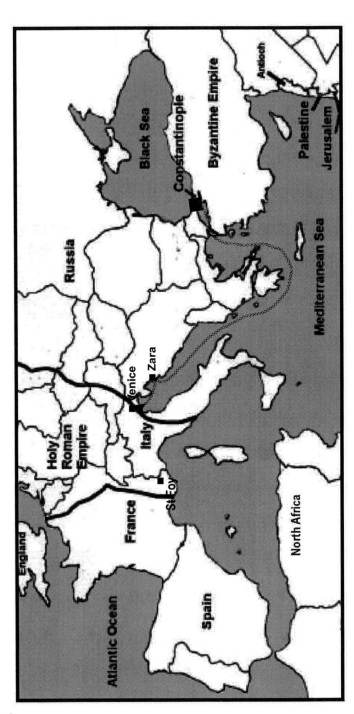

The route of the 4th Crusade

~

Part One

~

O GOD how am I to tell this story, this story of the second betrayal of Christ and the desolation of the greatest and most beautiful city in Christendom?

I am the Prioress of St. Foy, a religious house in the province of Lyonnais and I would keep the silence of my Order but for a voice that cries out to be heard, the voice of a child now dead to the world. She was there and it is her story I must tell.

Kitty is the common name for a common infant left in the porch of our priory. She was found by a nun who carried her to the altar, called her "the little Christian" and left her to the mercy of God. Luckily, the child's cries were heard by the old cleaner, who took her to the hovel where she lived and brought her up in the ignorance and dirt of her occupation. "The little Christian" became Kitty, a plain girl with a round peasant face, brown eyes and freckles, strong from scrubbing the stone floor of the chapel and stupid either by nature or neglect. Her fate was decided, she would scrub floors and grow old quickly and die, until God intervened in the person of His representative on earth, the Pope Innocent III. We are often the victims of the ambitions of great men. If there ever was an innocent it was Kitty. She was twelve or thirteen, she could say her Paternoster and Ave Maria without knowing a word of what they meant and she was as born a victim as any lamb.

It was the Good Friday in the Easter of the year 1202. Robert of St. Foy, whose father had built the priory to celebrate his return from the last disastrous crusade, led his family and their retainers past the old man's effigy in full armour lying on his tomb, up to their places of honour on one side of the altar. What they lacked in fortune they made up for in pride. They looked askance at God on their right and the wretched people on their left, bare-headed and many bare-footed, shuffling into the chapel. It was small and served by only a few old nuns, with the peasants and their families huddled together like sheep. Last and least was Kitty in her smock of raw wool, squeezed in by the door and pressed against the stone stoup of holy water on the wall.

She could hear little, the drone of the priest reading St. John's description of the Passion of Christ as if it was a schoolboy's Latin oration. She could see little, only the backs of the people bowed by labour more than reverence and above their heads the gilded feathers of the ladies of St. Foy nodding like their wearers. The heat and the stink of sweat and incense made her head spin, the shades of childhood fell from her eyes and for the first time she became conscious of her insignificance, her wretchedness, her hopelessness. She realised of all the misery in the chapel she was the most miserable. She owned nothing. She was nothing. No one would want her as a companion let alone a wife. No one would take the trouble to speak to her, even to insult her, or beat her, or crucify her ... someone was preaching, not in Latin but in her own language.

"These are not my words. These are the words of God, the words of Christ Himself. Christ is here standing among you."

The people stirred and looked about uncertainly.

"Christ is standing here weeping. His wounds are still bleeding. Christ's blood is falling on you."

There was an audible groan and a woman cried out. Kitty strained to see who was speaking, but she was too small to see over the heads of the people.

"Christ has been brutally cast out of His Holy City, the city made holy by the blood of Christ. Christ is suffering. Take pity on Christ."

They knew about being cast out and they took pity in their murmured prayers and cries.

"Jerusalem, Christ's city, has been captured by a host of foreign unbelievers. They have despoiled the holy places and Christ's Sepulchre, the holiest place in Christendom. The sacred Cross, the true Cross stained with the blood of Christ, is in the hands of heathen men."

The speaker's voice trembled with passion. The people had never heard anything like it before and it reverberated amongst them.

"Our Christians in the Holy Land are hemmed in, in the cities of the coast. Christ calls you to go to them and with them to go to Jerusalem, to take back Jerusalem for Christ, to become soldiers of Christ, to join the army of Christ, to take up the Cross of Christ!"

Now there was a general outcry and movement amongst the people and Kitty was able to push between them and stand on the foot of the font to see the pulpit and the small black-garbed monk under its canopy.

"There will be dangers. A hundred years ago your forefathers faced dangers and overcame them and captured Jerusalem, Jerusalem which now has been wrested from them by the paynims. But where there are dangers there are rewards."

Here was something new for the people. Pope Innocent knew his people.

"Whoever takes the Cross and confesses will be given absolution for all his sins and when he dies, in whatever country, he will receive eternal life in the hereafter. This man will not be cast into Hell and every sin, no matter how deadly, will be forgiven."

He promised Heaven and the people were only too ready to accept it. They pushed forwards towards the altar, much to the peril of their lives on earth. Kitty stood staring into some unimaginable future.

"There are rewards in this life also." The monk's voice had an edge of cynicism. "The Holy Land is full of riches, wealth and lands flowing with milk and honey. There are riches for today and the promise of Heaven for tomorrow for all who take the Cross in the army of Christ, in the army of God."

They raised their arms like children in school. They gaped as fish gape when they take the hook. Their eyes were bright and their heads were full of hope.

"The Holy Pope Innocent has called for a new crusade! Take the Cross! Take the money and land! Take eternal life! O God, who will not fight for Christ where he lies bleeding? Remember it was done for you!"

Now my lord's retainers had to link arms to protect the St. Foys from the enthusiasm of their subjects. Robert stepped down and went to the altar followed by about a dozen men, servants, tenants and some strangers Kitty had never seen before. The black-garbed monk had left the chapel, doubtless to go on to the next one and the local priest, Robert's brother Aimery, stood before them. They knelt.

"Do you swear you will go to the Holy Sepulchre in Jerusalem under arms?"

They swore it, muttering the words. He took a handful of white ribbons from the altar, each embroidered with a red cross and placed them on their shoulders.

The men replied, "Lord bless this sign of the Holy Cross and let it aid the salvation of thy servant."

Aimery warned them, "You have sworn before God to go on this pilgrimage. Remember, only His Holiness the Pope can now dispense you from your oath."

If those who had sworn had any doubt they did not show it. If they had known the truth of this crusade they would have damned the Pope and gone to hell anyway. At the moment they were heroes. Robert rose and led the men out with his family and all the rest cheering and shoving through the narrow arch of the doorway - all except for Kitty who had the floor to clean before the midnight Mass.

On her knees, dragging the wooden bucket after her, she was in a turmoil of longing and fear. The black-garbed monk had spoken to her, appealed to her, for the sake of a man more wretched and miserable than she was. He had begged for her help. She longed to go to his aid and that was her fear. How could she help him? She was only Kitty.

As she washed the floor, the dying sunlight lit the painted saints on the walls of the chapel. They had died for Christ. The old crusader's tomb stood like a rock in the shadows and the sculpted skeletons on the base danced the dance of death. Above the altar hung a wooden screen newly painted for the festival with a Christ crowned with thorns hanging on the Cross watched by St. Mary and St. John. The work was naïve, distorted by a clumsy hand, but in the glimmer of the dying candles on the altar it had a horrible reality. The painted blood dripping from the five wounds had not yet dried and crept down the Saviour's thighs. Kneeling, Kitty looked up and saw a miracle. Christ Himself was begging her for mercy. Her child's heart leapt for him and she was lost.

A slanting ray of sunlight illuminated a corner of the screen where, as in the pages of a missal, stood golden cupolas and silver towers within the walls of a city. It was Jerusalem. Kitty saw the Jerusalem of her dreams and in that moment poor Kitty became a crusader. A few of the white ribbons were lying on the altar. She stood up and took one and laid it across her shoulder, the red cross showing. She knelt. The great resolve burgeoned in her heart and she whispered, "I swear."

She never knew the nun who had given her to God, but now she was God's.

In the days that followed, the people of St. Foy were busy preparing for the departure of Robert and his troop for the Holy Land. Kitty watched them with excitement and the inner thrill of her secret plan to follow them. Horses were brought in from the fields for the few privileged to ride them, carts were requisitioned to carry their arms and provisions. The blacksmith worked overtime to sharpen their swords and lances. The rest, retainers, peasant farmers, vagabonds, wore their own clothes and bore home-made pikes and axes. The strangers Kitty had seen in the chapel appeared to be armed already. She had no thought of taking anything more than herself to defeat the enemy and capture the Holy City on her own. She had made one decision, to become a boy. The old cleaner had a son who had left her as soon as he could walk the distance to the next town and Kitty took the few rags of clothing he had left behind. Her hair was kept short to deter the lice that infested the hovel. She had no thought of what might happen in the future. She had no thought at all.

As the time of departure came nearer, the excited activity in the town lapsed and a gloom descended on St. Foy. People remembered how few of the men who had gone on crusade with Robert's father had returned. There was the long journey by land and sea to the Holy Land, the dangerous campaign against a fierce enemy, the old lord had said that the Saracens fought like Christians and there were the perils of thirst, hunger and disease. They knew they would not see their menfolk again for two years, if ever.

On the day, their spirits rose again. Bells were ringing, drums were beating, a colourful parade marched from the castle of St. Foy down through the town on the road to the east. Kitty watched them excitedly in the unthinking and delightful anticipation that she would soon be joining them. Robert and his brother Aimery led the procession on horseback, their gaudy surcoats emblazoned with their crest and the badges of the minor nobility to which they were related. Their pages followed in a cart decked with ribbons and their masters' shields and lances flying gay pennants. Their retainers wore their master's livery and all had the ribboned crosses on their shoulders. The people cheered, forgetting this panoply had been paid for by their industry and their indigence. The peasantry recruited from the land straggled afterwards with their makeshift weapons and well-worn jackets and smocks, but all were cheery and smiling, as if to say they would not have to work tomorrow. The strangers were in a group at the back and they were cheered though no-one knew who they were or why they were going on crusade.

As the tail of the column disappeared from sight, the gloom returned. The people drifted back to the fields and workshops. Their toil and struggle would only be ended by death.

Where was Christ in all this? He had been forgotten.

That night, Kitty put on the boy's clothes and stole out of the hovel. The old cleaner was sleeping in her bed by the fire. She had never been kind, but she had never been cruel. Kitty turned and whispered, "God bless you." Christ had not been entirely forgotten. Then she ran away from St. Foy, barefoot and almost as naked as when she had entered it. Christ was in her heart and His Holy City in her eyes.

But I forget. She is no longer she. She is a boy.

~

Part Two

~

OWARDS evening on the second day the boy came up with the troop camped on the banks of a river. Robert's pavilion was pitched in a field of flowers that rivalled in colour his heraldic gauds. His black horse cropped the grass and his retainers were busy preparing his dinner. It was the smell that drew the boy on.

He was nervous that someone from St. Foy would recognise him and he waited until dusk. The smoke of camp fires drifted up from the companies encamped all along the river, which was full and fast from the melting snows in the mountains. The boy thought they would only have to cross the river to reach the Holy Land.

When it grew darker he approached the camp. He crossed the rim of light from the first fire and stopped dead. The strangers he had seen in the chapel were sprawled around it. They started up and he saw the glint of steel. There was a suckling pig on a wooden spit above the fire that kept him from running away.

A fat man, who in better times might have been a bishop, muttered, "It's only a boy, come here boy." He moved into the light. "It's a hungry-looking boy. What are you doing here boy?"

"Sir," the boy had learned the hard way to be polite, "I'm going on the crusade."

They laughed. He took the white ribbon from his shirt.

One of them said, "He stole it." And another, "He's in good company then."

The bishop spoke quietly, "What's your name, boy?"

"It's Kit, sir."

"Come to the fire Kit. Are you hungry, Kit? Can you cut up a pig for … how many, Kit?"

"Seven, sir."

"Eight, Kit, eight." The bishop turned to his flock. "He's one of us, my friends. He'll look out for us, won't you, Kit?"

There was the hint of a threat in his voice. Kit turned and knelt by the fire. He poked the pig with a stick. "It's almost ready, sir."

He trusted them. They were crusaders, sworn to God. They ate the pig and went to sleep. He lay on the ground with them. He was happy. He slept.

In the morning, Kit could see the extent of the army gathered by the river Saône. Camps stretched in both directions as far as he could see. They were waiting for barges to come downriver from Lyons to carry them across, though the wisest among them were saying that the current was too full and fast for the barges to move at all. Days went by and Kit stayed with his new companions, fearing to go among the men of St. Foy and be recognised. He fetched their firewood and their water, he cooked the pigs and chickens that mysteriously appeared, he washed their clothes when they became over-infested with lice. From their rough jocularity and camaraderie he thought they liked him. Once he asked them their names. They had eaten and were throwing dice and passing round a flask of wine when he came back from wiping the dishes clean on the damp grass.

"What are your names, gentlemen?"

They whipped round and stared with suspicion.

The bishop spoke. "Have you been talking to someone?"

"No, I want to know your names so I can pray for you."

They laughed with relief.

"Oh pray for us Kit, but we have no names. We are like brothers in a monastery. We have occupations."

"You're a bishop, sir, aren't you?"

"Indeed I am, but it's a secret. The others can speak for themselves."

"I am a lawyer," said one. "A merchant." "A soldier." "I am a gentleman, a member of the noble house of Guise." "I'm a poet."

The last to speak was a small rabbity man, smarter and cleaner than the rest, who either had no occupation or one he could not even lie about and all he said was, "Deuce."

It finally dawned on the Generals commanding the army that the barges were not coming. There were two main contingents, one from the provinces and lordships of the north and the other from those of the south. The north decided to march to Lyons and cross the bridge there and the south decided to do the same at Vienne. Lyons was in the north and Vienne was in the south, so they both went back the way they had come. They had wasted three months of summer.

They met again at the foot of the Alps.

There had been an incident at Vienne which had puzzled Kit. It was taking an age for the cavalcade to cross the narrow bridge. He and his companions were last as usual, as if the tail was somehow the best place to be. Suddenly the one who said he was a poet appeared at his side and pushed a bundle of clothes into his arms. In his surprise he dropped it and a pair of boots fell out onto the cobbles. The poet picked them up and pressed them on him.

Kit asked, "Who?"

"From your Uncle Flyn," said Poet and disappeared.

Apart from the boots there was a pair of leather breeches, an undershirt and a coat of fleece. Kit took them into the camp that night.

"Very nice," said Bishop, "Where did you find them?"

"I didn't." He glanced at Poet, who ever so slightly shook his head. "Uncle Flyn gave them to me."

They laughed. "You never told us you knew Uncle Flyn."

"I don't."

"Of course not, none of us do, do we gentlemen?" They laughed again and shook their heads.

"Who's Uncle Flyn?" His innocence amused them.

"Only the greatest thief in Ireland," said Bishop.

Nothing more was said about the gift except when Kit remarked he never wore boots.

"You will, boy, you wait when you get up in the mountains."

There were the mountains. Kit had seen them in the distance for the last week and they did not seem so terrible, but now they were higher than the clouds. His only thought was that the Holy Land was on the other side. His feet were entirely innocent of boots, but they were soon familiars.

Up and up they climbed into a cerulean sky, until night - and then it was only Uncle Flyn who kept him alive.

The long trail of men dragged itself upwards until it reached the pass of Mont Cenis, where the wind roared and the ice never melted and then blissfully down into the merciful plains of Montferrat and Italy.

"Is this the Holy Land?" Kit asked Poet.

"Ah, Kit, Kit, the only Holy Land is the one we left behind us."

He was Irish.

They marched on day after day. It was late summer and no-one had told them where they were going. Some said to Rome, some to Genoa, it was all the same to Kit. He was going to Jerusalem. The sun shone, the harvest ripened, there were pigs and chickens in the barns and plums and peaches in the orchards, there was wine in the taverns and there were women everywhere. Crusaders knew they were already forgiven for their sins by the oath they had taken.

Once, Kit got a glimpse of the Generals. The army was camped on the slopes above a city. A horde of traders had arrived to take their money and one of thieves to steal it. The tents were scattered over the fields like daisies. Kit was looking at the smudge of the city in the distance when the man who called himself Deuce came up and sat next to him.

"That there is Turin," he said.

"Have you been here before?"

"No, no!" Deuce hunched his shoulders as if to hide a secret.

There was a disturbance behind them and they saw a bright and shining cavalcade, armed and beribboned, men and horses in chain mail and cloaks of velvet laced with gold, long steel-tipped lances like maypoles, the whole glittering pageant trotting between the rows of tents.

"Nobs," said Deuce.

The riders spurned the shabby shelter Kit had built for his friends, the horses snorted and rolled their eyes, the great men at the centre of this galaxy disdained to look at the two creatures sitting on the ground.

"You see the crosses on their banners," said Deuce, "they mark their companies so their men follow them and no-one else. The red is for Count Louis of Blois. The blue, Count Hugh of St. Pol. Yellow, Baldwin of Flanders, more important than the others. Green, the Marquis of Montferrat himself, the Emperor's cousin and the Pope's best friend."

"How do you know?" asked Kit.

"Oh, I don't," said Deuce.

Shortly after this, Deuce disappeared.

The march eastwards was resumed through the long days of summer and the lush landscape of Lombardy. Kit had been struck by Deuce's acquaintance with the world and wondered whether the other companions could enlighten him. Soldier was the oldest and had seen service in the last crusade. He was also the quietest and had seen more than he wished to say. Kit polished the old man's dented helmet, round and shallow like a surgeon's bowl and gave it back to him. Soldier looked tired. His long face with his drooping nose was grey and his eyes were dim and deep-sunk in their sockets. He put the helmet on his grizzled scalp but not before Kit had noticed a long scar like a furrow in a winter field.

"What was it like sir, the crusade?"

The old man did not answer.

"Did you know the lord's father in St. Foy?"

"Maybe," said Soldier.

"Did you go to Jerusalem? Did you see the king of France?"

"He run off and left King Richard on his own." He was English.

"Where were you wounded? Why are you going back?"

Soldier looked at Kit with eyes that had seen too much.

"Nowhere else to go."

He looked back into a past he could not bear to see again.

They marched on past hills and lakes and peasants harvesting in the fields. The sun hung low and the days grew shorter. Winter was in the offing and where were they going?

"To the Holy Land," said Kit.

"Yes my dear, but how?" replied Bishop.

"By land," said Lawyer.

"Only a fool," replied Merchant, "you'd have to pay the Greeks and fight the Turks to get there. By sea!"

"Can't swim," said Poet.

"We're going the wrong way," added Soldier.

They all looked at Gentleman who had not been listening.

He jumped.

"My cousin is distantly related to the King of Albania," he said.

"Yes," said Bishop, "that's why you've got no boots."

Kit had a happy thought. He was better off than the King of Albania's cousin.

They marched round a lake as big as a sea and onwards, keeping to the country ways, the column straggling for a mile or more, avoiding the towns and cities because the Generals feared crimes and desertions. Kit discovered that a soldier sees little more than the back of the man in front of him, learns little more than how to steal and feels little more than his feet. Jerusalem and the bleeding feet of Christ were memories. The cause was lost in the practice.

They marched into autumn and the rain-soaked plains of the province of Veneto. They were sodden, their clothes rotted on them, the dye ran on the ribbons on their shoulders, looking like a raw red wound.

Deuce reappeared.

"Venice. We're going to Venice."

"Is that near the Holy Land?" asked Kit.

"It's on the sea. We're going on the sea."

"There's ten thousand of us," said Bishop, "and horses."

Soldier spoke. "Five hundred men or fifty horses in a transporter. Some of the horses died and some of the men. We sailed from Marseilles."

"Is that near the Holy Land?"

Soldier turned to Kit.

"You wouldn't be so eager, boy, if you knew."

"Milk and honey," said Poet.

"Blood and plagues," said Soldier.

On the march again, Deuce dropped behind the others to where Kit was struggling with their paraphernalia and relieved him of some of it.

"I went to Rome. I heard something. Have you heard anything?"

"No," said Kit.

"About a treaty between the Generals and the Venetians?"

He was not a very good spy because he asked the one person in the army who hardly understood a word he heard and then forgot it anyway.

"No," said Kit.

"There was one about a year ago. They were going to pay the Venetians a lot of money to take us in their ships to Egypt."

"Is it near the Holy Land?"

"No it isn't. Egypt is the richest place in the world."

"Why do they want to go there with an army?"

Deuce piled the pots and pans back on Kit's shoulders and marched on disdainfully.

That night they were lying under Kit's awning around a smoking fire, steaming like cattle come in from the cold, when the boy suddenly asked the man nearest to him, who happened to be Gentleman, why he had come on crusade. Egypt had stuck in his mind.

"Me?"

"Was it for money?"

The others were watching. Gentleman was offended.

"I despise money. I took the Cross because it was expected of me. For honour. For glory. I admit there was a lady in the picture, but for honour, boy, for glory."

"Were you running to her bosom?" asked Bishop innocently, "Or running from her husband?"

Gentleman rose with dignity.

"You are unaware of the code of chivalry," he said and walked out of the shelter. He returned a moment later.

"It's raining."

He sat down, pulled his ragged coat around him and rubbed his cloth-bound feet.

"He should go and see Uncle Flyn," said Kit.

The army marched on and then suddenly there was the sea. Kit had never seen the sea and the flat grey strip between a brown landscape and a gloomy sky was not impressive. He did not realise it was the sea until Soldier came up and said, "Horrible."

"What?"

"The sea. Horrible."

"Why?"

"If she turns bad there's no escape. You can run away and hide on land."

Kit wondered if he had.

"The sea," said Merchant that night, "is the lifeblood of commerce. Some of my best deals were done at sea."

"You spent a lot of time on land then," said Bishop.

Lawyer, who seldom spoke for nothing as if he were still in practice, remarked that the sea was a good source of litigation.

"A clever man can make his fortune without leaving his chambers."

"Money," said Gentleman, "all you talk about is money. We didn't take the Cross for money, but to right a great wrong done to God."

God had hardly had a mention since they had left St. Foy.

Kit suddenly saw the congealing blood creeping down Christ's thigh. He felt a flood of shame and embarrassment rushing through his veins and he called out, "Christ's blood!"

They were taken aback as if their own crimes had caught up with them.

Bishop muttered, "That's right. No thieving when we get to Venice. No taking the money out of people's pockets, no stealing their victuals or their fine linen, no cutting of purses."

He looked benign and innocent, but his darting eyes and a little twist of a sneer betrayed his delight at the prospect of eating his own words.

In fact, they never got the chance. The Generals had agreed with the Doge and Council of Venice to take the whole army by barges across the lagoon to the island of St. Nicholas, a long sandy spit a league away. Only Poet was pleased, he could not think of a rhyme for Venice.

St. Nicholas nearly finished them. The island lay between the lagoon and the sea, without trees or vegetation and the only building a monastery. Looking out, Kit could see the masts of a great fleet of ships, like bristles on a hedgepig, on the rim of the lagoon and imagined they would soon be taking them to the Holy Land. He returned to the shelter to find Bishop and the others grumbling about a lost opportunity to rob the Venetians and how to rob their fellow crusaders. Strangely, the Generals had the same problem.

About a week after their arrival, a company of Sergeants went from tent to tent demanding a silver mark from every man to pay his passage. Of course when they got to Kit's shelter he was the only one there. He had never seen a silver mark let alone owned one. The Sergeants had no roll of names, nor would the strangers' names have been on it, so they left the boy but not before one of them took him out into the light to have a look at him. Kit knew from his livery that the Sergeant came from St. Foy and began to tremble.

"Are you ill?" asked the Sergeant.

"No sir."

"Wrap yourself up lad, this is a desperate place."

"When will we go to the Holy Land, sir?"

"When the Generals have got enough money to pay Venice to take us. Half the army's not come."

Kit told the others when they had sneaked back after dark.

"I wish I hadn't come," said Merchant.

They had a fire of driftwood and some dry beans stolen from the provisions supplied by the Venetians. Kit boiled them in dirty water.

"Why did you come?" asked Bishop.

"I suppose it doesn't matter," said Merchant, "we'll all be dead soon. I was swindled by my partner over a cargo of goods he said was sunk at sea, but I know it wasn't and the goods were landed somewhere and sold. I was ruined and had to leave the country."

"You should have taken him to law," said Lawyer.

"He took me."

"It's always the way," Bishop nodded wisely, "do as you would be done by."

"I'm not the only one." Merchant looked at Lawyer.

"My case was entirely different," Lawyer looked offended. "I was appointed by the Court to defend the leader of a gang of cut-throats and they threatened me with death if I didn't get him off. He was as guilty as Judas and I had to flee or flout my conscience."

"What happened to him?" asked Kit.

"Somebody bribed the judge and he got off."

"Before or after you fled?" Bishop smiled innocently.

Lawyer was silent, but Soldier spoke.

"I fled. At the battle of Hattin when Saladin took Jerusalem."

He said no more and the others looked away not to see his shame.

Gentleman broke the silence.

"I come from a great family and a small estate. I had only one thing to do with my life, to marry a wealthy woman who would exchange her money for my name. I couldn't do it. I loved a young lady with the love the minstrels sing about, but she was forbidden to me because she was my brother's daughter. She had a beauty and spirit that put all other women in the shade. When she was of age my brother brutally married her to a man of no name but great wealth, but when she had no children he put her aside. She became wild and reckless, wasted her settlement on fools and rascals. She refused my help and shortly after she died in poverty. I swore to Christ, if He would take her to a better place, I would take His Cross."

Kit's eyes were wet and he said it was the smoke from the fire.

Poet spoke next.

"I also have a love that will not die. She too is beautiful, wild and wilful, at once as young as spring and as old as winter. The west wind is in her hair and the sun behind the clouds is in her eyes. She is the jewel in the sea, the emerald in the ring on a king's finger, she is my mother and my sister and my lover. She is Ireland."

There was a moment before they all looked at Deuce, who stood up and said, "I've got to go outside."

Bishop spoke.

"I suppose I must. Well, my friends, I was a priest, not a bishop as young Kit believes but a parish priest and I served my Saviour faithfully for many years. One day, the Bishop came to my parish in all his pomp and splendour, his lackeys rode palfreys while I went on foot, his belly was big and his face shone like a kettle. He admonished me for my poor appearance, declined my offer of hospitality and hurried back to his palace. I decided I would live like a bishop. You know the Church sells sin in the form of indulgences, forgiveness at a price. I turned the confessional into a shop. This went well, everyone sins and pays for it, but I over-indulged and with the profits I became a profligate. Women, wine, whatever. I outdo you, my friends, whatever you do, I've done more often."

"But why take the Cross and march across Europe and be stuck here on this midden?" asked Lawyer.

"Gold, frankincense, myrrh, whatever's going," said Bishop.

"What about the Holy Land? What about Christ?" Kit's shout startled them.

"When you grow older you'll understand," said Bishop.

"Then I shan't grow older!"

"Not if you go on like that!"

From that evening onwards Kit mistrusted them. He felt ashamed of them and awkward in their company. Fortunately it did not last long. One dark day that spelled winter, the Sergeant who had quizzed him appeared and ordered him to come at once to Robert of St. Foy's pavilion. Kit thought he had been discovered and tried to run, but the Sergeant seized him by the arm and dragged him out. This predicament was seen by the others and they shook their heads and congratulated themselves that it was not them. "I had great hopes of him," said Bishop, "he'd have made a good thief."

The Sergeant marched the wretched boy across the sands, past tents where crusaders sat like crabs cold and hungry and waiting for the tide, to the rising ground on the island where the great men had their pavilions as gaudy as a fairground.

Robert's pavilion was small but comfortable, with a stove, a cot, a prie-dieu chair on one side of which he could kneel and on the other sit, where he was writing at a table. The Sergeant thrust Kit in front of him.

"Here's the boy, my lord."

Robert barely looked up.

"He'll have to do. How is Simon?"

"Worse."

"Get the boy washed and dressed. I have to attend Count Louis within the hour."

Washed and dressed? What for? Kit feared that it might be for his execution, or worse, the dress might be a dress and he would be exposed for what he really was. He had not thought about it until then.

The Sergeant took him to the officers' latrine, a luxury he had not experienced before. At one end there was a tub and a pitcher of water. He left Kit to wonder what it was for and returned a few minutes later with a page's uniform.

"Aren't you washed yet? Get in the tub! Take your clothes off first!"

Kit peeled off his coat, his boots, his breeches and stood in his undervest which reached to his knees.

"Get in! You can wash that, too."

He climbed into the tub. The Sergeant poured the pitcher of cold water over his head and left him shivering. He got out at once and looked at the clothes the Sergeant had brought. There was a clean vest, drawers, undershirt, silk breeches, stockings, shoes, a warm tunic and a tabard embroidered with the blazon of St. Foy, a sable falcon on an azure field. He dried himself on his old clothes and put on the new. He immediately felt nobler. The Sergeant fetched him, smoothed his hair and put on a velvet cap with a feather.

"Come on, cupid."

Robert was waiting with his Squire. He looked once at Kit without a flicker of recognition and led them down to the shore to join the exalted company of the great lords Montferrat, Baldwin, Louis and Hugh and their entourage. A barge took them to a Venetian galley lying offshore and they were rowed swiftly across the lagoon towards the city.

Hundreds of ships were moored in the lagoon, fighting galleys, transports, ships with a ramp specially adapted to carry horses and the Doge's own rich vessel coloured vermilion like a poppy in a field of corn. Kit wondered at this vast armada and what it was meant for. To take them to the Holy Land of course.

Venice by comparison looked dirty. The seafront was a long brown line of warehouses and shipyards, offices and counting-houses. The Doge's palace stood out white and behind it the domes of St. Mark loured over the city like rainclouds. That was all he saw because the landing-steps led directly to the palace, the great men went inside and he and a few other pages were left loitering on the wharf by a stinking canal.

Venice was made for money. The few Venetians Kit saw were stony-faced greedy-looking gargoyles who looked remarkably like each other. He asked one of the pages, "Are they talking about money?"

The boy, who served one of the Counts and hardly deigned to speak to a mere lord's page, replied, "Money is for miscreants. Haven't you heard of chivalry?"

"There was a horse in the village."

They laughed at him and turned away. They bore the arms of France and the Holy Roman Empire on their tabards. The deputation came out of the palace with an old white-haired man wearing a conical hat and fur-trimmed coat and they stood on the steps arguing about money.

The crusaders still owed half the sum they had agreed to pay Venice. Two-thirds of the army had failed to arrive, either sailing from other ports or reneging on their vows to take the Cross, or falling sick and perishing on the march. The Doge of Venice, the old man in the conical hat, was insisting they should be paid for the great effort and expense of building the fleet, while the Generals were protesting they had not got the money. The Doge threatened to starve the men on St. Nicholas and the Generals warned that starving men become desperate. They had moved away from the Doge and Kit saw the old man was still talking and realised he was blind. Montferrat returned and touched the Doge's arm. They walked aside, whispering to each other. Montferrat came back smiling and Baldwin, Hugh and Louis lifted their heads and nodded enthusiastically.

On the trip back to the island the word passed from mouth to mouth, Venice had agreed to put off the debt until it could be paid from the profits of the crusade. Kit wondered what profit could be made from Christ.

The boy feared he would be sent back to the gang of thieves. Simon the page recovered and Kit had to return the livery. He was given instead a woollen suit and a leather apron and told to report to Lord Robert's farrier as he would be working in the stable. His first close sight of the warhorse Thunderer made him wish he had been sent back. The great black heavy horse stood as tall as Kit and half as much again. Thunderer was built to carry a knight in chain mail from head to toe, bearing a shield and couching a lance as long as two men. In battle he wore his own chain armour and headpiece and was caparisoned from feathered hoof to flowing mane. He looked at Kit with blue-brown eyes and thought he would do.

He did. Thunderer went from walking the boy to allowing him to sit astride his massive back and encouraging him to trot, canter and one day gallop along the strand, kicking up the waves. Of course, Kit thought it was the other way around. Above the world he found a new freedom, the spirit of the wind and the sea and the great horse infused in him a life beyond the life he knew, like the moment in the chapel and another moment he would one day experience.

He was grooming Thunderer when someone sidled into the stable and stood in a dark corner and hissed.

"Kit, it's me. Are you alone?"

It was Deuce. He shuffled warily around the horse.

"Here, you know everything, where are we going?"

"We're going to the Holy Land."

"That might fool the others but not me. You're in with the nobs now, you can tell me."

"You said it was Egypt."

"No, the Venetians have done a deal with Egypt. I don't trust them. Neither does the Pope."

"How do you know, Deuce?"

"Oh, I don't."

Thunderer turned his head to look at Deuce. He did not like him.

Kit asked, "How are the others?"

"Fine. The gentleman's dead of a fever."

"He's with his love," said Kit, "he took the Cross so now he's in Heaven."

"No he isn't, he's under the sand with a stone on top of him. Kit, I've got to find out where we're going."

"Come with us and you will."

When it was announced that they were going to embark, the crusaders, who had spent three miserable months on the island, made bonfires of the last of the driftwood and ate the last of their wretched rations. They cheered the lords who were about to deceive them. Indeed, Montferrat left the camp almost at once. They sharpened the weapons they had been using to chop wood, wore their crosses once more with pride and waited agog to learn where they were going. All except Kit who was sure he knew.

The boy was getting Thunderer ready for battle, a familiar procedure for a horse trained in the tournaments at home, which were ruled by chivalry and fought with ferocity.

The ships in the lagoon began to manoeuvre nearer to the island. The narrow galleys with their oarsmen anchored offshore, while the shallow draught transports, broad- beamed between two raised castles, bumped against the sand so men could wade out to them. Kit counted up to ten and gave up, but there were twenty times that number of ships and they were taking twelve thousand souls and fifteen hundred horses on board in the service of Christ.

As part of the deal struck outside the Doge's palace, the Doge himself, Enrico Dandolo and some six thousand Venetians, took the Cross and joined the crusade. Only one of them knew where they were going and he was blind and silent.

As the companies boarded the transports bearing their lords' colours, the priests, who had spent the exile comfortably in the monastery, reappeared and mounted the castles to pray and they all sang the crusaders' hymn "Veni creator spiritus".

As Kit led Thunderer down to the strand to join the other horses, one was as apprehensive as the other. The huge cargo ship had a ramp cut out of the side which led to the hold, where each horse was boxed separately and haltered to keep it from panicking. The ramp was drawn up, the sail hoisted and the ship scraped off the sand and rolled out into the lagoon. As it seemed to float, the boy swallowed his fear and climbed up on the forecastle. Two hundred ships, the transports flying the colours of their counties and provinces, the galleys' gunwhales lined with the shields of their lords, the Doge's vermilion flagship and the Venetian vessels proudly decked with the banners of St. Mark, slowly sailed out of the lagoon and into the Adriatic sea.

Kit spent most of the next three weeks in the box with Thunderer. He avoided the other grooms with their games and stories. He had a fear of company and had only endured being with Bishop and the gang because they had accepted him without question. He dreamt of a Jerusalem with golden cupolas and silver towers in the corner of a hill that bore the Cross of a suffering Christ. He had no notion of how Christ had lived or what Christ had said, only that Christ had suffered and died on the Cross. It was the injustice that fired his soul, the rest would come later.

The fleet made steady progress along the Dalmatian coast, keeping the land in sight. Winter was no time for taking to the open sea in shallow craft. The boy had no sense of time. It was the cessation of movement and the rattle of the anchor chain that told him they had arrived.

He ran to the deck and climbed up to the forecastle. The fleet was standing off a harbour with the entrance barred by an iron chain suspended between two buttresses. In the shadow of the hills beyond lay the grey walls and towers of a city. Kit's instant disappointment was tempered by the thought that Jerusalem, being by the sea, was somewhat tarnished. The other grooms were shouting and pointing and he saw a Venetian galley heading towards the entrance of the harbour at speed, the oars oscillating like the legs of a beetle. They watched with growing excitement as it crashed into the chain and the iron prow of the galley snapped it as if it had been cotton. Anchors were raised and sails loosed and the transporters were shepherded into the harbour by the galleys like sheep into the fold.

Kit said to the boy next to him, "That's Jerusalem."

It was the one who had twitted him in Venice.

"Idiot! It's called Zara. It used to belong to Venice, but they rebelled and now we're going to get it back. You were there at the Doge's palace, that's when they did the deal. They get Zara and we sail to the Holy Land in the spring."

He turned away with the double satisfaction of his superiority and generosity in enlightening a fool.

The Venetians landed and camped on the open ground opposite the city. The Doge's red tent was the centre of attention and Kit wondered how Enrico Dandolo, old and blind, was so powerful.

He had to learn that power itself is old and blind.

The orders were given for the crusaders to disembark and prepare to besiege Zara. The pavilions of the great lords were pitched near that of the Doge and Robert's was one of the nearest. His Squire and the Sergeant laid out his weapons and armour and all the colourful trappings a knight bore into battle. Kit did the same with Thunderer, who stamped his huge hooves and snorted with excitement. Kit could see the Doge's pavilion and remarked the series of incidents that followed. The Generals Baldwin, Louis and Hugh came out of the pavilion and returned to their own quarters. A deputation arrived from the city, soberly dressed elder citizens of Zara, who doffed their caps and bowed their heads as they entered. Then the Doge himself came out with his secretaries and hurried to the Generals' headquarters. A white-robed monk and two crusader lords, who might have been waiting for this moment, went in.

They came out shortly afterwards with the whole Zaran deputation which hurried off towards the city. The Doge returned with the Generals, walked past the monk and his companions and entered the pavilion. Then they came out and angrily confronted them and there was a fierce argument in which the monk waved a letter and Lord Baldwin waved another. Robert appeared from his pavilion and ordered Kit to get on with his work.

Somebody hissed behind Kit's back.

"Is that you, Deuce?"

Deuce came out of the shadows with Bishop and Lawyer. Bishop was wearing some rusty scraps of armour over his leather jerkin and Soldier's helmet on his head and Lawyer, rather incongruously, carried a spear.

Kit asked, "Is there going to be a fight?"

"Oh yes, my son," said Bishop, "there's going to be a fight and there's going to be prizes."

"How do you know?"

"Deuce here heard it all. He was in the old man's tent."

"In the privy," said Deuce, "I was sitting there so no one could come in."

"Go on," said Bishop, "tell him."

Deuce took a deep breath.

"First comes the old men from the city to see the Doge and they say spare us and we'll open the gates and let you in and Enrico says it will cost you dearly but we'll see no one gets hurt. They say God bless your honour and he says I've got to tell the crusaders because there's more of them than us and he goes off to talk to them."

"I saw that," said Kit, "and then a monk and two lords went in."

"That's right," said Deuce, "he said he was the abbot of somewhere and he swore we wouldn't fight against a Christian city because there was a letter from the Pope forbidding it. The Pope wrote, 'Don't attack a Christian city or I'll excommunicate the lot of you,' or something like that and he showed them a copy."

Kit was puzzled. "What Christian city?"

"That one over there," said Bishop.

"Well," continued Deuce, "the old men were laughing and cheering and they all went out."

Kit added, "They went back to the city. We can't attack them now. What did the Pope say he'd do?"

Lawyer butted in. "Excommunicate, cut you off from the church, no christening, marrying, burying, no confession and absolution, no Heaven, boy, no eternal life."

"Is that what Christ wanted?"

"What's that got to do with it?" asked Lawyer. "Anyway, the Pope had already written another letter which was nailed to the church door before we started."

"Count Baldwin had a letter in his hand," said Kit.

"It's a handy letter," Lawyer smirked, "the Pope wrote that we weren't to attack any Christian city, but listen, boy, unless they impede the journey or there is a just and necessary cause."

"There isn't, is there?" Kit asked.

"I'm a lawyer, there's always one."

"If we want to go to the Holy Land we've got to pay the Venetians," said Bishop, "and if we want to pay the Venetians we've got to help them take Zara, besides, once we're inside we can give them a good sacking."

"That's what they were arguing about. The old Doge was furious and the abbot kept crossing himself, I watched them through the loophole. Then someone knocked on the door and I had to get out."

Deuce was disappointed.

Bishop put his arm round Kit. "Join us when the siege is over and I'll make you rich for life."

Kit wriggled out of his grip. "You're wearing Soldier's helmet."

"He doesn't need it any more Kit. He's dead. We buried him at sea."

"He hated the sea," said Kit.

When they left he did not follow them.

What did the two letters from the Pope mean? One gave them permission to do anything necessary to reach the Holy Land and the other forbade them to do the one thing necessary to get there. Kit was too young and stupid to realise the Pope wanted the crusade to succeed at all costs and at the same time did not want to be accused of condoning an outrage against Christianity. In the Church, the end justifies the means. In Christ, the means are the end.

The siege of Zara lasted five days. The citizens hung crucifixes and Christian banners from the walls, but it did not stop the Venetian warships closing and projecting heavy rocks from their siege engines at the same walls. The crusaders assaulted the walls from the land and dug trenches to undermine them and bring them crashing down. On the sixth day, another deputation of elders came to the Doge's pavilion to surrender the city and beg him to spare the lives of the citizens. The gates were opened and the two armies rushed in to break down doors and steal the contents of the houses and churches, which they later occupied for themselves and their horses. There were murders after dark. It was a year and more since they had left their homes, marched through snows and storms, starved of food and expectations. Time enough for them to forget their vows and remember their vices.

Kit entered Zara with Robert's company. Thunderer galloped away, the men scattered in search of booty and he was left in a mêlée of Venetians and crusaders fighting amongst themselves for scraps. He ran away and hid under the galilee of a monastery. The iron-studded door was bolted and the few looters who tried it gave up. Kit saw a monk running towards the monastery and suddenly Bishop rushed out of an alleyway and struck him down. What did a monk have that Bishop wanted? Then he saw Bishop strip off the monk's habit and put it on over his jerkin, pull the hood over his helmet, clasp his hands together and approach the monastery. He hammered on the door until a wicket opened and a monk peered out. Bishop cried, "Sanctuary, Brother, sanctuary!" Kit heard the bolt being withdrawn, the door opened and Bishop went in. The monk Bishop had struck had not moved and Kit was frightened to follow him. He waited until Bishop came out without the habit and patting his jerkin, bulging and clinking with stolen treasures.

Kit entered the monastery. The nave was dark, with strips of winter daylight piercing the lancet windows. He tripped over something black and saw the body of a monk. He felt sick. He had eaten with Bishop. He walked along the nave to the altar. The cloth had been swept aside and a silver candlestick still stood, too big to steal. The paten and the cup had gone, stuffed into Bishop's jerkin. Kit was leaving when he saw a glint of gold, a crucifix with a golden Christ had been flung aside. He picked it up and saw Bishop had tried to wrench the figure from the cross and failed. Kit held it and remembered that on the rood-screen in St. Foy Jerusalem had been golden and Christ had been naked. The whole purpose of the crusade seemed to have been twisted like the figure on the Cross. Christ was poor, had nothing, asked nothing. What was the purpose in going to Jerusalem? To seize the Holy Sepulchre? Christ was not there. To seize the wooden Cross? Christ was not on the Cross, any more than Christ was on the cross he held in his hand. It became worse as he realised Christ was not on the painted screen in St. Foy and the blood was not Christ's blood but his because it was in his head. Why were they going on crusade? To redeem Christ or to regain the kingdom of Jerusalem, the gold the preacher had promised for those who went? What did men worship, God or gold? Bishop worshipped gold, perhaps bishops do as well. What do I worship, he thought. He had come a long way from St. Foy and had even longer to go to God.

The epidemic of looting burned itself out. The Generals decided to spend the rest of the winter in Zara, dividing the city with the Venetians and taking the best houses for themselves. The plan to use the money and treasure to settle the debt to Venice and sail for the Holy Land in the spring failed. The Venetians, claiming the sovereignty of Zara, took the lion's share, the lion was the symbol of St. Mark. The crusaders squandered or hid the rest in their scrips. When winter was over, there was not one silver mark in the kitty more than there had been when they came to Zara.

Kit was quartered in the fine house Robert of St. Foy had seized for himself. He felt more comfortable with Thunderer in the stables. Each morning they exercised on the shore. The sandy beach was usually deserted, but one morning he saw someone he recognised wandering through the dunes. It was Poet. Kit rode up and Poet crouched down and cried, "Don't kill me, I'm a writer!"

"Poet it's me."

"Is that you Kit? What are you doing on that black monster, have you stolen it? I had a silver piece and I took it out here to hide it and now I can't find it."

"I saw Bishop," said Kit, "how are the others?"

"Ah, my boy, Merchant's happy buying and selling stolen property and Lawyer's defending the one man the authorities have charged with theft. Deuce has gone again."

"And Bishop?"

Poet wriggled uneasily as if the answer had to be twisted out of him like a cork from a bottle.

"The same but worse, Kit. He calls himself Lord Bishop and lives in a monastery hearing confessions and selling indulgences. Will you believe it, he's holding services for christenings and marriages and funerals, which we can't have from our own priests because we're excommunicated by the Pope!"

"How are you, Poet?"

"I live in comfort, but comfort doesn't suit me, Kit, it's want what makes me write."

Kit laughed, but Poet was serious and added, "You don't want to get to Jerusalem, it's not what you think it is."

Kit had the same thought in the monastery. Poets have a way of telling the truth.

The year changed. The winter was unchanging and the crusade was on the beach at Zara. Venice had agreed to supply the fleet for a year and half of it had gone. The Holy Land was still the goal, to redeem the vow they had taken and fight for the Cross, win or lose and make their peace with God and man. Jerusalem was as far away as ever.

Kit learned a soldier's life is mostly soul-dulling tedium, the repetition of pointless tasks until he becomes desperate to go into action, to live or die but at least live first.

There was a stir of interest when the Marquis of Montferrat arrived back from Rome with a delegation of serious-looking Germans and the pronouncement that His Holiness the Pope was remitting the sentence of excommunication. He had accepted their contrition for attacking their fellow Christians on the doubtful axiom that when war is waged by God's will it is a sin to doubt its righteousness.

Robert of St. Foy was summoned almost daily to attend his overlord Count Louis of Blois at the conferences held by Montferrat, the Germans and the Generals. Thunderer was in and out of the stables with Kit holding the stirrup for his lordship's foot. He saw from Robert's face that the life of a great man was not without the same cares, conflicts and tests of conscience that plague paupers.

The problem was obvious. The crusade could go neither backward nor forward. Some lords and their companies were already leaving to make their way to the Holy Land as best they could. The rest were discontented with their leaders, in spite of the preacher's promise, they had neither money nor salvation.

Then it leaked out that Montferrat had brought a solution to the problem. The Germans were part of it, the Pope was behind it and the Doge, old blind Enrico Dandolo, was very much in favour of it. What it was, nobody else knew. Kit expected Deuce to come and ask him, but the thickets of diplomacy were too dense even for spies.

Weeks passed, the days lightened, the small enamelled flowers that herald spring appeared and the Venetians began demolishing the walls and buildings of Zara, leaving only the churches standing. The crusade was on the move again, but where was it going?

In April 1203 the fleet sailed away from Zara, carrying almost half the number of crusaders who had left their homes a year ago. Death, disease, desertion, delay and despair, had whittled away the battalions that had set out to save God and their souls. Those that remained were bound by their oaths, or poverty, or lust, or the inertia of a soldier's life, stuck between idleness and duty.

Kit was standing on the quay, watching the sails disappear. Thunderer had gone on a transport with the long-suffering endurance of an animal trained by man. Kit would have cried, but he was part of a Guard of Honour, Robert of St. Foy, his Squire and his Sergeant, his Page and his company. Simon was ill again and was being sent home on the Roman galley they were expecting. In his stiff tabard and tight breeches, Kit thought crying inappropriate. Two Venetian galleys lay in the harbour, waiting to carry them in pursuit of the fleet with their mysterious guest.

The Roman galley, too shallow, round and cumbersome to keep up with the fleet, wallowed into sight, rowed by unwilling slaves. It was high in the water and a single plank had to be lowered from the deck down to the quay. Two men carried Simon's litter precariously aboard and then they waited for the promised saviour of the crusade to appear.

A young man clad in foreign clothing, a light silk coat, silk culottes, all in beige, curled shoes and curled silky dark hair, tripped down the plank like a ropewalker and posed for a moment on the quay. Kit thought it was a woman until he saw Lord Robert kneel to kiss the young man's jewelled hand. The Squire and the Sergeant knelt and Kit gathered that this was expected of him and would have done so but for the breeches. Instead, he bowed as far as the tabard would let him and hoped he would not be noticed.

He was, but not for the discourtesy. He dared to look up and saw the face of a Madonna, oval, olive, dark eyes full of laughter or, as Kit saw later, tears. The jewelled hand was there, not to kiss, but to raise Kit's face to the stranger's and then was gone. Kit felt something he had never felt before, his heart beating.

He did not see the young man again until they were at sea in the leading Venetian galley. He asked who the young man was, but the Squire was silent and the Sergeant only knew that he was Greek.

"Watch out for Greeks lad, they've got bad habits."

Two days out, the sail was spread and the sun was shining. It was early morning and Kit lay on his back on the foredeck. Before he could jump up, the stranger signalled him not to move and sat on the deck beside him. He spoke with a soft, strange accent, without any respect to the grammar.

"Forgive me, I am Greek. Do you speak Latin?"

Kit shook his head.

"Then I must do my best. What is your name?"

"Kit, my lord."

"Call me Alexius, while we are on this boat call me Alexius," he paused and smiled down at Kit, "and I shall call you Eros."

He lay next to the boy, not touching but so close Kit could feel his presence.

"This is my last chance to be a man before God makes me an emperor." Kit could not talk.

"Speak little one. This is what I feared, no-one will speak to me again except to tell me lies."

They lay silent in the sun until the Squire appeared and stared at them with horror.

"Your Highness! Your breakfast, Sire."

Alexius sighed and rose like a cat and left them.

"How dare you! You'll be whipped." said the Squire.

Kit was not whipped but called to Lord Robert's cabin.

"I don't know who you are, but I suppose you belong to me and I'm responsible for you. This young man is the son of the emperor of Byzantium. Well, he was the emperor until he was deposed by his brother but that's no affair of yours. He's a great man and we have plans for him, do you understand? Don't talk to him. Kneel when he comes in. For Christ's sake do like the rest of us!"

Strangely enough it was for Christ's sake.

Kit did not dare to go above deck for the rest of the journey. The Sergeant watched him and the Squire, who liked Simon, scowled at him.

Corfu was a Greek island, a part of Alexius's empire if he ever won it, but the small population showed no enthusiasm for his arrival. They satisfied themselves by throwing a few stones at the crusaders and selling them their produce at a profit. The camp was set up in a bay sufficiently far from the principal town to avoid trouble. There was nothing to do for God's army but to lie in the sun and watch the horses grazing in the spring fields, completely unaware their futures were being bargained for above their heads.

Alexius was escorted to a pavilion between those of Montferrat and the Doge to keep him under surveillance. The Germans had gone home having come to terms with the Generals. Kit was reunited with Thunderer. They were on a hillside some distance from the camp. Kit was lying on his back in the sun and Thunderer cropping the carpet of spring flowers. A rider on a horse from Montferrat's stable approached them and Kit recognised him and jumped up before remembering to kneel.

"Not here Eros. Not yet."

Alexius was wearing Turkish trousers and a blouse. He dropped down with a sigh.

"They talk all night. I offer them all they ask, all the German emperor's people agreed. He is married to my sister. Still they will not sign."

He raised himself on one arm and gazed at Kit.

"What terms will you agree?"

Kit was in a whirlpool of emotions he did not understand, as if they belonged to someone else, which in a way they did. He was a boy, but did boys have these feelings?

"Tell me, Eros, are two hundred thousand silver marks enough for you? And provision for your army for a year? And I will raise ten thousand men for your crusade and come myself? No? Shall I promise to bring the whole Greek church in obedience to Rome and make Pope Innocent supreme patriarch of the world? Yes if I have to, to become Emperor."

Alexius rolled onto his back and Kit, glancing at him, saw tears in those dark eyes.

"Don't cry my lord."

"I will not if you will call me Alexius. I cry for justice. Justice against the man who put out my father's eyes and took his empire for himself, his own brother, my uncle. Justice for a crime against his sovereign appointed by God, against God."

Justice for Christ! The feelings that had overwhelmed Kitty in the chapel arose again in Kit. He wanted to comfort Alexius, to hold him, to offer to give his life for him and might have done so but a sudden ice-cold awareness of who he was stopped him.

He was Kitty and Alexius believed he was Kit!

The young man, who was old in experience, knew the difficulties and rewards of innocence. He sat up and bent over Kit, his madonna face close, his ringlets caressing the boy.

"Do you agree?"

He would have done if he had been Kit. He would have done if he had been Kitty and Alexius had asked Kitty and not Kit. As it was, he said nothing.

Alexius knew if he sprung the game it would spring and he would not catch it. He sighed.

"We have so little time. Be here tomorrow."

Kit was there with Thunderer the next day and Alexius rode up from the camp.

"All they do is argue between themselves. It is simple. We sail to Constantinople, the people rise up and kill my uncle and declare me emperor. I meet the terms of the agreement. We sail for the Holy Land and capture Jerusalem. Why do you not speak?"

"For Christ, take Jerusalem for Christ, not for you."

"Constantinople is my Jerusalem. Have mercy on me, Eros."

The appeal reached Kit's heart and a spring of love filled his eyes. He longed to touch Alexius, but then Alexius would touch him.

Kit loved but could not love. It was a torture devised by the devil as a punishment for loving Christ.

Alexius did not stay. The boy was impossible. It was true.

As he was riding back to camp Kit saw Bishop haranguing a group of crusaders. When they saw Lord Robert's horse they scattered. Bishop looked dejected.

"Ah, Kit, I wish we'd never left Zara."

Kit asked after the others.

"Merchant's gone. He cheated too many men as was safe to go out in the dark. He slipped off in a boat going to Marseilles to cheat at home. That rascal Lawyer's gone over to the other side."

"I'm sorry he's dead," said Kit.

"I wish he was. He's joined the Provost Marshal, damn him. He knows too much about me. I'm sick of this crusade."

"And Poet?"

"He's no use to me. He couldn't steal a ducat from a blind man."

Kit thought it might be some sort of fowl.

"I'm going home, lad."

"Your oath, Bishop, in the chapel, to redeem Christ."

"Each to his own. If Christ wants to be redeemed, let him redeem himself."

"Jerusalem."

"Every man's got his own Jerusalem, Kit and mine isn't surrounded by sand and full of foreigners."

Kit was determined to make Bishop do the right thing to make up for all the wrong ones.

"We might not be going to Jerusalem."

Bishop was interested. "Have you heard something?"

"We might be going to a place called Constantinople."

"Constantinople? I love it!"

"What is it?"

"All the money in the world." Bishop was in the heaven of his heart.

"And we go to the Holy Land after." Kit reassured him.

Back in the stables grooming Thunderer, Kit heard a familiar hissing behind him.

"You can come out, Deuce."

Deuce emerged from behind the manger.

"I saw you talking to Bishop. Don't trust him, Kit."

"I don't. I saw him knock a man down in Zara."

"Only one? Here, tell me everything you know."

It would not have taken long but Kit was busy with Thunderer.

"You're a close one," said Deuce, "I knew it when I first saw you. I knew you were hiding something. What about the Greek gentleman?"

Kit ducked under Thunderer to hide from him.

"Well, I'll tell you. He wants to be emperor of Constantinople and the nobs are arguing should we help him or not. Montferrat and the Generals say yes because he'll give us a lot of money and almost everyone else says no because we should be in Jerusalem by now."

Kit thought of Alexius.

"We can go to Jerusalem later."

"With a lot of money? I doubt it."

"Don't you trust anyone, Deuce?"

"It's not in my nature," said Deuce.

When the crusaders learnt of the bargain the Generals had made with Alexius, the greater part refused to accept a scheme that would subvert their oaths and divert them from God to mammon. These simple men had more faith than money. The final confrontation between the Generals and the army took place outside the camp in a valley where the leaders of the

Jerusalem party had retreated. Montferrat, Baldwin of Flanders, Louis of Blois and Hugh of St. Pol rode out with Alexius in a desperate attempt to save the crusade. Robert attended Louis and Kit ran at his stirrup to hold Thunderer later. They dismounted in front of the nobles and knights who had pledged their word to God, of the priests who were in horrible fear of the Pope and of the thousands of simple men who had given up their families and occupations and were ready to sacrifice their lives for Christ. Watching, Kit was torn between his love for Christ and his love for Alexius.

Then he saw the Generals, great men who ruled counties as large as countries, kneel before their liegemen, their tenants and their serfs and beg them to accept the undertaking to which they had already put their names. They swore it was the only way to save the crusade, that Alexius would be received with joy by his subjects and the army would be in the Holy Land before the end of summer. The dissidents held a conference and returned to declare they would go to Constantinople on the condition that they would stay no longer than a month and then would sail for the Holy Land. They all swore on the Gospel, wept and embraced, except for Kit who did not know whether to laugh or cry.

At the end of May 1203 the crusade embarked on the Venetian ships and set sail for Constantinople.

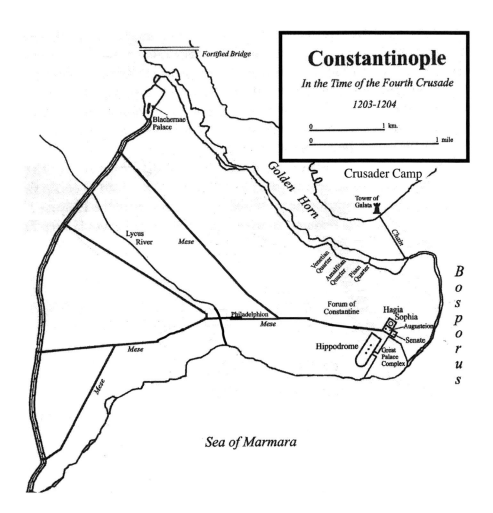

Fortified Bridge

Constantinople

In the Time of the Fourth Crusade

1203-1204

0   1 km.

0   1 mile

Blachernae
Palace

Crusader Camp

Golden Horn

Tower of
Galata

Lycus
River

Mese

Chain

Venetian
Quarter

Amalfian
Quarter

Pisan
Quarter

B o s p o r u s

Forum of
Constantine

Hagia
Sophia

Augusteion

Philadelphion

Mese

Senate

Mese

Hippodrome

Great
Palace
Complex

Mese

Sea of Marmara

~

Part Three

~

HIS WAS not a city, Kit thought, it was a world. The walls were as high as hills and the towers along them unscalable peaks. From the lighthouse marking the entry to the Bosporus they stretched as far as he could see, like the mountains barring the route to Mont Cenis. Beyond the walls he saw thousands and thousands of roofs and rising above them palaces, domed churches, the arches of a vast amphitheatre, statues and triumphal columns and above them all the huge golden dome of a cathedral mothering a cluster of smaller domes like a clutch of eggs, thought Kit. He was watching from the forecastle of the horse transport, almost the last in the procession of the fleet, dressed overall in shields, flags and banners as, after a month at sea, it came into sight of Constantinople.

Enrico Dandolo, Doge of Venice, had taken over the conduct of the campaign partly in deference to his age, which Kit had heard was ninety and more so in relation to his experience in dealing with the Greeks. He knew the strengths and weaknesses of Constantinople, which had dominated the seas for ages and which Venice envied with all its heart. He led the procession in his gaudy galley past the city close enough to the walls for the thousands of Greeks crowding them to marvel and throw stones, beyond the headland that led to the inlet called the Golden Horn which separated the city from the mainland, to land on the opposite shore near the small town of Scutari.

The crusaders made camp under the colours of their lords and walked about after a month at sea. Kit settled Thunderer and walked to the seafront to gaze at the city that was not Jerusalem. It appeared more formidable than ever, the walls were higher and it was defended on both sides by water. The entrance to the Golden Horn was blocked by a chain between towers on both ends. He knew they had come to support Alexius's claim to the throne in return for money and men enough to take the crusade to the Holy Land. What would they do if the Emperor of Byzantium politely refused to abdicate in favour of his nephew? Sensibly he put the question behind him, that was the business of the great men who had brought him there and then, being stupid, he thought they could answer it.

The Emperor did what Kit expected. He had brutally betrayed, blinded and imprisoned his brother and he probably thought that the same would be done to him by his nephew. He wrote to the Generals to ask them why they were there, he offered to provision the army until they left for the Holy Land and warned them that he had received a letter from the Pope in which His Holiness had told him he had forbidden the crusaders to attack another Christian city. Innocent was protecting his innocence.

To emphasise his determination, the Emperor ordered a display of the enormous power at his command. Kit heard a discordant blare of trumpets and the thunder of drums in the distance. The crusaders ran from their tents and the Venetians crowded the sides of their ships. Looking across the Bosporus they saw the huge gates in the walls of the city open and a stream of soldiers pour out onto the ground between the walls and the sea. Battalion after battalion formed up in an array glittering with the sun catching on pikes and spears, swords and axes. The battlements bristled with archers armed with crossbows. Huge wooden engines, mangonels and petraries, capable of hurling great rocks an arrow's flight, rolled forward on the tops of the towers. In the city every rooftop in view was filled with citizens and on a mound of rising ground a horde of armed militiamen was assembling.

Lord Robert's Sergeant was standing near Kit and reckoned there were a hundred thousand soldiers and as many as five hundred thousand militiamen and he had been in the last crusade.

Kit asked him, "How many are there of us?"

"Maybe ten thousand, boy, but remember they're Greeks and numbers don't count." He might have been a politician.

"There aren't any horses," said Kit.

"They don't need horses to defend a city and we don't to take it, horses can't climb walls. But let them come out and we'll show them what they can do. They're only Greeks."

Somebody murmured, "They beat the Persians at Salamis and three hundred held the pass at Thermopylae against the whole Persian army."

"Different Greeks," said the Sergeant.

Kit recognised the murmur, "Poet?"

The Greek army began retreating into the city and the crusaders returned to their tents. Kit and Poet stayed in thrall at the spectacle of such threatening magnificence, or so Poet said.

"I'm enthralled by the spectacle of such magnificence," said Poet.

"I wondered where you were."

"Ah, Kit, I'd have been somewhere else if I could. What are we doing in Constantinople?"

"We're going to put Alexius on the throne and then we're all going to the Holy Land."

"So that's it. I'm better for that."

"You're laughing."

"I'm laughing at swearing an oath at St. Foy to do one thing and finding myself here doing another, like we did at Zara."

"This is for Alexius."

"It's not for Christ, that's sure."

"It's for justice, Poet."

"Sure it is," said Poet, "to tell a foreign party what to do and kill him if he doesn't do it and then we go back home."

"It's so we can go to Jerusalem!" Kit's voice was shrill.

"Did you see the men's faces when they saw the golden city? Did you see the riches shining in their eyes?"

Kit cried out, "Am I the only one who believes in Christ?"

"No," said Poet, "but you're the only one who thinks it's going to happen in this world, in this time, Kit, in this way."

"What are you going to do, Poet?"

"I'm going to die for the wrong reason," said Poet, "don't you."

In order to redress the balance of power, the Doge decided to show Prince Alexius, as he was now called, to his people. Kit wanted to see Alexius again. He had decided to tell him the truth that he loved him and rely on

Alexius's love allowing him to overlook the slight flaw in Kit's make-up. The Doge's galley was moored in the harbour at Scutari. Kit settled Thunderer and ran down the hill to join the crowd waiting to see the pretender. Venetian sailors forced a passage to the galley and the Doge was carried aboard in his chair. Kit heard a few people cheering and, fearing he would miss the hero, pushed to the front and peered between two guards. Alexius wore a purple robe and the red silk stockings which were the prerogative of Byzantine royalty. Long curls framed his angelic face and Kit thought he looked like the young Christ. Alexius mounted the gangway to the foredeck of the galley. Kit tried to follow him but was thrust aside by the sailors. He ran along to the stern where the rowers were boarding on a plank leading to the lower deck, went among them and managed to reach the long dark gallery lined with wooden benches and crossed with shipped oars. He hid behind one of the broad rough-cut ribs of the ship, though the rowers would hardly have noticed him. They were the able-bodied detritus of society which makes up most of the world, unchained but slaves nevertheless to poverty, intolerance, unemployment, persecution, depression and failure. They were the convicted and the convinced that Christ would save them, if not in this world then in the next. The man who died on the Cross was one of them and so they wore His cross, just like their lords and masters pacing the deck above their heads.

In his chair on the foredeck Enrico Dandolo had convinced himself that the appearance of Alexius would spark an uprising in the city, or at least a palace revolution. It is the discontented nobility, those nearest the throne who have been disappointed or cheated or cuckolded, who get their revenge at night with a dagger and then proclaim the rights of man. So the Doge put Alexius on the prow of his galley, raised a flag of truce and set off across the Bosporus with ten galleys in attendance. When they were in shouting distance a herald declared, "This is Alexius Angelos, your rightful emperor," several times and the curious Greeks who had gathered on the parapets shouted back, fortunately in Greek so that Kit in the hold did not understand them. The galleys rowed up and down almost touching the walls only to receive a barrage of boos and jeers and laughter and, from those who bothered, stones. The Doge sent a priest up the mast to preach that God required them to displace the usurper and crown the true emperor and behold there was a priest on top of one of the towers preaching that God would destroy the invaders unless they went away. This is what the crusade had come to out of necessity.

On the way back to Scutari, the Doge, as vermilion with anger as his ship, had himself carried to his cabin. Alexius, as red with embarrassment as his stockings, sat alone on the foredeck, watched with a trace of contempt by some sailors in case he threw himself overboard. Kit saw his chance to come up on deck and nobody stopped him this time. He did not realise the extent of Alexius's humiliation, the height from which he had fallen. Everyone from his royal relatives to the Generals and the Doge had assured him he would be received in Constantinople with acclamation and declared emperor by popular consent. His own vanity was broken like a mirror and perhaps that is what hurt him most. Kit approached the quivering back of his lover and knew he was sobbing. He hesitated and then put his hand on the purple shoulder. Alexius sprang up, saw the boy and all his fury at himself and the world burst out in a cry that brought the sailors running to him. He stared at Kit with such hatred that the madonna turned into the medusa and Kit was turned to stone. The sailors dragged the boy away and threw him back into the hold, where he stayed until the galley docked and he dared to creep down the gangway.

The Sergeant was waiting for him.

"You," he said, "are going to be hanged."

Kit did not mind.

Lord Robert had ordered Thunderer to be saddled and made ready. They ran to the stable and Kit bridled Thunderer, the Sergeant threw on his saddle and Kit tightened the girth. They pulled his cloth embroidered with the black falcon over his croup and led him out to run as fast as they could to the lord's pavilion. Robert had no time to swear but trotted off with Kit hanging on to the stirrup to the field where a council of war was being held. The Generals remained mounted whilst they planned the campaign where they would not be overheard. The grooms were gathered together in a corner of the field.

"What's going on?" asked the smart one.

For once Kit knew more than he did.

"They laughed at Prince Alexius and threw cabbages and other stuff at us."

"We'll have to beat them now," said the smart one.

He was right. The crusade could go neither backwards nor forwards without provisions and money to pay the Venetians and the only money was in Constantinople. The vast wealthy Christian city with its enormous army stood between them and Jerusalem. They were soldiers and their heavily armoured cavalry was invincible in open ground, but useless in the siege of a city. Kit heard the Generals intermittently as they worked out their strategy. The walls abutting on the Bosporus were too close to the water for an assault by land. There was a good space between the walls and the Golden Horn, but the mouth of the inlet was guarded by a chain strung between two towers. They could land on the mainland, but then they would have to cross the Golden Horn with men and horses to reach the city. Someone asked what the Venetians would do and Robert, the least important member of the council, said, "Let them land us and from then on it's our business." War was the only business of a gentleman. His ancestors had won his land and titles by force of arms. He had practised fighting mock battles and in tournaments, which had a practical purpose apart from entertainment and a display of chivalry. A crusade was as necessary to his honour as it was to his soul.

It was not so to Kit and the common man. The word that they were going to assault the great agglomeration of walls and towers and the vast army awaiting them across the water led them to line up to seek the priests, who heard their confessions, gave them absolution and assured them the cause was sacred, sanctified by the Pope and would take them to heaven, sooner or later. Kit had his mission from Christ and nothing to confess.

Action banished fear. The foot soldiers, who were clad as they had come from feudal farms and the poorer parts of towns, sharpened their makeshift weapons, axes and pikes fashioned from the blades of their scythes fastened to poles. The archers and crossbowmen, professional hunters and fighters, put on their padded leather jerkins and round helmets, honed their arrows and re-strung their bows. The sergeants, who were mounted on wagon horses, each wore a hauberk and their lord's colours on their pikes. Lord Robert's Sergeant wore a black falcon on an azure field. Robert himself was protected by chain mail from head to foot, a hood and cape, a hauberk and breeches, covered by a surcoat blazoned with his device and a cylindrical helmet with slits for eyes and mouth. He fought on Thunderer with a lance or on foot with a sword, perhaps his father's, whose stone sword measured from his chest to his feet. Kit carried the sword and Thunderer had his own coat of chain mail from head to tail and hanging over his legs to protect him from his only vulnerability, being hamstrung. So the crusaders prepared for war.

The Venetians were not idle. The Doge, perhaps stung by being excluded from the planning, was also eager to take the opportunity to attack an old enemy. The Venetians' element was the sea. They mounted siege engines on the towers of the transports and piled up heaps of rocks and stones. Their crossbowmen were stationed on barges, which the galleys would tow together with the transport ships across the fast-flowing Bosporus. The Doge was determined to play a principle part in the assault and win a large share of the subsequent rewards of victory. He had a plan of his own.

Early on a sunny morning in June 1203 Kit was woken by a reveille of trumpets and drums, the call to arms. He hurriedly equipped Thunderer and led him out to join the parade of horses heading for the harbour. The crusaders marched in their divisions to where the transports were waiting. At these moments every man is wrapped in his own thoughts. Kit was fearful now that death was a possibility for himself, for Thunderer, for the Sergeant, for Poet, even for Bishop. He saw Bishop in the ranks of men and Bishop saw him and amiably waved with the large axe he carried on his shoulder. Kit wondered if he could kill a man, he knew Bishop could. Would it be for Christ? What use would it be to Christ? Or if he was killed what use would that be? He did not want to die for Alexius. Yet if it was not for Christ it would be for Alexius, to make him emperor. If it was for Christ he would go to heaven. If it was for Alexius it was doubtful. He was being jostled and squashed in the press of horses and grooms pushing to mount the ramp of the transport. Thunderer was bucking and trampling and he was hanging on to the reins and it struck him that he was likely to be killed in the next minute if he did not stop thinking.

One by one the galleys drew the transports out of the harbour to join the fleet which covered the sea. They slowly moved out into the Bosporus towards the mainland. Kit saw Constantinople as a moving panorama, the great grey walls banded with red bricks, the many domes of the churches, the towers, the golden bowl which he had been told was St. Sofia, though he did not understand what that meant and pouring out of the gates in a glittering torrent an army coming out to meet them. Kit thought that the Generals knew what to do.

The Generals, meeting on the Doge's flagship, had no idea. They had never planned a seaborne landing before and they had not now. They looked at each other for an answer and finally at Robert of St. Foy who had boasted, "Let them land us and from then on it's our business." They turned to the Doge. Enrico Dandolo smiled, an old man's smile that said I've done it all before and said nothing.

The passage to the mainland against the current was slow and when the leading galley came within bowshot of the shore the vanguard of the Greek army was already deployed against them. Dandolo raised a hand and the barges were released to move forward and swing sideways to face the enemy. The Greeks started to shoot arrows at the barges, but nothing to the arrows that came in return, as if a dozen hives of bees had been disturbed and were taking their revenge. The vanguard fled back to the large body of foot soldiers waiting cautiously out of range. The galleys hauled the transports up and as they bumped against the sand the soldiers leaped out and waist-deep waded to the land and formed their ranks. The ramps were lowered and the grooms ran into the sea with their horses and Kit, who never set foot in water without a shudder, was nearly drowned as Thunderer charged splashing to the shore. The lords and their squires in armour were rowed in barges from the galleys, but even they were too keen to meet the enemy to wait and waded ashore to climb up on their steeds and take their lances from their squires. They rode to the front of the ranks, a steel-clad line of death.

If an army can tremble, the army of Constantinople trembled. Behind their ramparts they were heroes, but with nothing between them and a charge of Frankish knights in armour there was no choice but to run. It was not cowardice but plain common sense. They had come from the city by a bridge over the head of the Golden Horn and the bridge would not have saved them if the crusaders had charged. The Doge and the Generals reasoned the precipitous retreat might provoke a rebellion in the city against the emperor and so the advance was no more than a gentle trot to chase the last man off the mainland. If there were any dead, they would have been killed in the rush to the bridge. There were a few who were robbed as usual and the Sergeant remarked they were not Greeks at all but mercenaries from the colonies of the vast Byzantine empire.

The crusaders camped on the ground they had taken. A council of war was held, this time in the Doge's pavilion out of respect to the blind old man's sagacity. Lord Robert was summoned and Kit followed in his train in case he was sent back for Thunderer. After about an hour Robert came out and addressed them, the Squire, the Sergeant, the Page and Kit.

"We're to have the honour of leading the attack to take the tower." It was his reward for boasting at the last council.

"Which tower, my lord?" asked the Sergeant.

"That one," said Robert, pointing towards the mouth of the Golden Horn.

It was dusk. Light from the beacons on the walls of the city flickered in the water of the inlet. A haze of light floated over the city that filled the horizon and the towers were black against it in every quarter. Robert was exasperated, it had not been a good council.

"That tower! The one this end of the chain! The Venetians want to bring their ships up here and attack the walls, you can't attack a wall from a ship! A ship is a ship!"

"The big tower?" asked the Sergeant.

"Yes. It's an honour. We've got a spy in there who says it's defended by what they call the Varangian Guards, Danish, English, no Greeks. Tomorrow."

The tower of Galata was the font of Kit's baptism in blood. In the morning the Sergeant mustered some fifty men, there had been near a hundred when they left St. Foy. Some of them had picked up weapons and armour abandoned by the mercenaries who had fled, but all of them would have been more at home behind a plough. Robert and his brother, Aimery the priest, rode up in full armour with their pages carrying their long swords. Kit followed Thunderer, to hold him when Robert dismounted to fight on foot. He had never felt such fear. There were ranks of crusaders behind them, but they were the forlorn hope, the desperate vanguard who would test the courage of the Varangian Guards. He looked round and was surprised to see Bishop among them. He had always thought that Bishop would be the first to arrive when the battle was over.

The march began along the shore of the Golden Horn towards the point where it flowed into the Bosporus. There was a cluster of mean houses dominated by a stone-built hexagonal tower, with an upper floor and battlements on the roof, standing next to a guardhouse. The chain that lay across the water supported on floats was anchored to the foundations. Every pace they took made it appear more ominous and impenetrable.

They marched into the sun with their pennants raised on pikes and lances. Their small numbers must have encouraged the defenders because when they came within bow-shot crossbowmen appeared on the battlements and a group of them emerged from the guardhouse. The crusaders were met with a volley of bolts, some of which found a mark and a man fell. Robert and Aimery raised their shields and rode on. Robert knew how long it took to wind a crossbow and load a bolt and reckoned they would take one more volley before they came in range of Thunderer. When it came, he spurred the great horse, who went into a trot and a canter and a gallop and Robert lowered his lance and charged the line of bowmen with Aimery beside him. The Sergeant cried out "Charge!" and the fifty broke into a run towards the tower and Kit came running after them. The most frightening sight in war is something coming straight towards you. The bowmen turned and fled but Thunderer was on them and they scattered. A few reached the guardhouse and ran inside. Aimery dismounted and before they could shut the door he jammed it with his body. God knows what blows he took, but he stood until Robert rallied his men and they pressed forward against the door and forced it open. Robert dismounted and followed. Thunderer was neighing and trampling the ground until Kit caught him and led him under the lee of the tower out of sight of the bowmen on the roof.

It was strangely quiet. Kit had readied himself for shouts and screams and somehow the silence was more terrible. Were they all dead? Suddenly Lord Robert appeared at an embrasure on the upper floor, white-faced and helmetless, crying out, "A sword! Get me a sword!"

Kit was petrified. Where could he get a sword? Only lords and sergeants wore swords. He looked round. The main force had halted five hundred yards back and the front rank was lined with lords and sergeants. He climbed up on Thunderer, whipped his head round and screamed "Charge!" Thunderer sprang off and charged straight towards the line of battle with Kit shouting, "A sword! My master wants a sword! For Christ's sake give me a sword!"

One lord more alert than the rest realised the boy was not mad and sent his page forward with a sword almost as long as himself. Kit hauled on the reins and Thunderer halted, planting all four great hooves in the earth, nearly shooting Kit off his back. Kit seized the sword, turned Thunderer and galloped back to the tower with the sword pressed to his body. He slid off the great horse and ran to the guardhouse.

There was a second before the sun left his eyes and he could see. Many of the bowmen were crouched along the walls, their crossbows futile in a little space and they were fearfully eyeing Bishop, who was walking up and down with his axe on his shoulder. Kit's instant thought was that he was calculating which of them had the most to steal. Bishop nodded at him genially and pointed to an arch leading to the tower.

About twenty men of Robert's troop were guarding prisoners in a stone room, apparently a kitchen, that took up the space in the tower. They looked almost as nervous as their captives and the nearest pushed Kit towards the stone steps leading to the upper floor.

The sudden darkness shocked him, his foot slipped and he put out a hand to stop falling. It came back covered in blood. His eyes darkened and he saw not steps but bodies tumbled and twisted with great wounds in their heads and shoulders, some of which heads he knew. It had been one-sided, there was not a single stranger among them. Grasping the sword, he had to climb over them. Some legs and arms still moved. There was light in the arch to the upper floor. It was a tableau-vivant, a still death. The room was divided by a long refectory table with benches on either side, scattered with plates and knives. First Kit saw the Varangian guardsmen on the far side, perhaps twenty Norse and Englishmen in iron caps and red leather harness studded with iron. They were holding long-handled axes, too long for the low-ceilinged room. On Kit's side, by the window embrasure, stood Aimery like a statue, the Sergeant, his pike levelled, the Squire with a short sword and Robert with nothing to strike with but his mailed fist. The poor Page was crouched nursing his hand which, Kit learned later, he had barked on the wall when he dropped the sword. Robert had turned his iron-clad head to see and grasped Kit's sword to go and stand by Aimery. The Varangian Guards had no weapons to pierce their armour nor had they the numbers to attack the Varangian Guards. Kit turned to the head of the steps and screamed, "A rescue! Come up!"

The first of Robert's men came up and stood beside their lord, then more until the numbers were even. One of the guards looking out of a window must have seen the main force of crusaders coming because he said something in a foreign language that made the others lay down their axes and kneel on the floor. They were sworn to fight to the death, but it is easier to swear than to die.

The crusaders cleared the tower of living and dead. Robert said nothing but Aimery patted Kit on the head as they rode off. The Sergeant came out of the tower dragging a wretched ill-favoured man by the collar. The man cried out, "Don't kill me, I'm a spy!"

"It's Deuce," said Kit, "I know him, he is a spy."

The Sergeant released him and Deuce and Kit walked back to the camp together. Behind them, the sappers were already striking with their picks to release the chain which eventually dropped and slipped into the sea.

Deuce seemed unaffected by his experiences and talked endlessly - most of the people in Constantinople were indifferent to who was emperor but only wanted to make money - the defences were strong but the army weak - the Pope was indignant but secretly delighted that when Alexius was emperor he would have authority over the whole Greek church and collect his pence from half the world - why did Kit keep rubbing his hand? Was he hurt?

It was the blood. Kit had seen death laid out in the chapel in St. Foy and it was the same as the carved death in stone and wood, but that death had a reason. What reason was there for the violent deaths in the tower? The feared Varangians were men and feared to die. What was death? The oath in the chapel had been taken by those who were dead and if God kept his word they would now be in heaven. What was heaven that it was worth the blood on the steps? Escape from hell. But hell was here and there was no escape from the axes of the Varangians. It was for Christ. Christ had died for what? So men could be hacked to death in his name? And those who killed them? Would they go to heaven when they were killed? Would Bishop go to heaven because he had taken the Cross? Or me?

Deuce was still talking.

"I have valuable information for the Generals. I wonder if they'll give me a shilling for it?"

The next four days witnessed a crisis in the campaign and another in Kit's life.

On the first day he was summoned to Lord Robert's pavilion. Robert was lying on his cot nursing his bruises. Though chain mail was virtually impenetrable it could only mitigate the force of a blow. Aimery was with him, his left arm wounded when he had thrust it into the doorway of the guardhouse. He was not wearing armour or his chasuble and looked fair, stout and handsome without them. He spoke first.

"What's your name, boy?"

"Kit, my lord." They were all lords to Kit.

"Kit, you're a very brave boy and I like that. I like the way you fetched my brother's sword. I like your bravery in the room with us."

Kit flushed. It was the first time in his life he had been praised, let alone liked.

Robert was less agreeable.

"That boy's no longer my page, you are. Ask the Squire for orders."

Kit was confused. It was a promotion but also a disaster, he would have to leave Thunderer. Robert barked at him.

"What are you standing there for?"

"My lord, Thunderer."

"Anyone can look after Thunderer."

"No they can't!"

Robert was astonished, as if no was an insult. He rose on his elbow. "Get out!"

Aimery moved between them. His nearness was impressive.

"Robert, the boy's right. No one can control that monster of yours. Who else could have ridden him so fast to get you a sword?"

"I've spoken," said Robert, "do you want me to break my word?"

"Never. He's your page. Send him to look after Thunderer."

So the feudal law was not broken, but Alexius's curse on Kit's emotions was. He returned to Thunderer and sat on an upturned bucket and thought of Aimery. How Aimery must already like him to defend him and then Aimery, Aimery, he loved the name, how long before he loved the man? Never! Aimery was a priest and unobtainable. Aimery loved Christ and Kit could not rival Christ. The passage between childhood and adolescence is as dramatic and perilous as the pass at Mont Cenis. Kit's childhood had been frozen, he had not broken the earth of the feudal society piled on top of him like a mountain. He had not known God except to scrub His floor. His awakening in the chapel had been an early spring, too early not to have been blasted by the frost of the world. His crusade had brought him emotions he did not understand, rejection and humiliation and disillusion, as it was continually being diverted away from the Holy Land to ends of greed and now power. Childhood is not innocent but it tends to be trusting. Kit was losing trust.

The next day the council of war met in the vermilion pavilion. Robert was not there but Deuce was in the privy.

"The thing about nobs," he told Kit later, "they stink just like us."

They were sitting on the ground outside the tent watching the sun shining aslant on Constantinople.

"It looks as if it's on fire," Kit said.

Deuce was unimpressed. "Enrico, he's the Doge, wants to bring his ships in here."

He waved at the Golden Horn, which by chance was golden at the time.

"He wants a couple of days to get them ready to attack the walls. The nobs all laugh and say you can't attack a wall in a ship and Enrico smiles and taps his nose with his finger and says nothing. The nobs think they've won and tell him how the army's going to march round to the bridge where the Greeks ran away and cross the water and attack the walls from the other side. Enrico says they've chosen the place where the walls are highest and they say he knows nothing about siege warfare and the higher they are the quicker they fall. Then he turns and says something in Italian to his friends and they laugh, the nobs get angry and demand to know what he said and he says he told them the walls will fall on top of them and he will be on top of the walls! They mutter among themselves about a stupid old man, I hear someone coming and have to get out."

Kit mused, "We're only a few thousand and they're ten times that."

"You don't want to talk like that," said Deuce, "someone might hear you."

That night as he lay on the straw mattress Kit thought of Aimery. How good he must be to love Christ and abstain from everything the world said was delightful. He was not sure what that was or that he had been deprived of it since his birth, but Aimery had renounced it and that made him a saint. In the warmth of Aimery's halo he fell asleep.

It was the second day. Kit woke and as he got up he saw the mattress was stained with drops of blood. He thought he could have squashed a bedbug and then, with more concern, that he had been wounded in the fight. The hand that had been bloodied in the tower was clean. He searched round the bed and suddenly noticed spots of blood on the undervest he wore. He quickly pulled it up and saw with horror blood trickling down his thighs. There was no cut, no wound, only blood on his thighs. He trembled before an explosion of enlightenment made him gasp. The blood was like Christ's blood in the chapel! He bled without a wound as Christ bled without a wound on the wooden rood screen and the wounded Christ bled on the wood of the Cross. It was a sign from heaven, the acceptance of his oath, the truth of the crusade, the echo of the crusader's cry, "Man have mercy on God!" His doubts were defeated and his questions answered.

The second council of war was held in the Marquis of Montferrat's pavilion. Deuce dawdled in the kitchen listening to their deliberations, whilst the Italian cook complained the chickens were scrawny and the onions soft.

"The old Doge sent his regrets," Deuce told Kit later, "and the nobs said they didn't trust him. I think it's the other way round. They said once he got his money he'd go home. If you ask me, they'll do the same."

Kit was indignant. "We're going to the Holy Land!"

"When?"

"When Prince Alexius becomes emperor and gives us the money to pay the Venetians we'll all go to the Holy Land. I know!"

"How do you know, Kit?"

Kit was silent. He would not betray God's secret.

He saw Alexius when he was riding back to the camp after Thunderer's hacking out. He was in a group of young crusaders with his arm round a fair-haired boy and a flask in his hand. He was drunk and dishevelled and dragged the boy into one of the tents. Kit tasted the bitterness of disgust. Men were going to die for that! How could he compare him to Aimery?

"How do you know, Kit?" asked Deuce with the persistence of a spy. It was evening and they were sitting in the usual place. The Golden Horn was full of Venetian ships dark on the water with the city looming beyond them. Five of the biggest transports had their masts stepped and the crews were active in the rigging, hauling up long balks and planks. They lashed the balks to the masts and laid the planks crosswise so that one end projected beyond the side of the ship. If the ship could sail close enough to the walls the planks would act as a bridge to assault them. It was protected by a covering of sailcloth and bowmen perched in the crow's nest above could shoot down on the defenders. Siege engines were being set up on the castles at both ends of the ships to hurl rocks at the battlements. This was the Doge's secret weapon which made him tap his nose.

"How do you know it's certain we'll go to the Holy Land?"

Kit was still silent. He had let the blood on his legs dry, fearing to wash it off might offend God. He was not going to tell his secret.

"You don't," said Deuce, "that's the answer."

On the third day Montferrat called a council excluding the Doge and he, Baldwin of Flanders, Louis of Blois and Hugh of St. Pol rode their chargers out of sight of the camp and out of hearing of spies. The grooms were below consideration. They were in a belligerent mood. They mocked the bridges the Venetians were erecting on their ships, flying bridges, a man would have to fly to get up the mast to cross them and if he did he would have to fight single-handed against the defenders on the wall. Their laughter sounded false to Kit and the accusation that the Doge would only pretend to help them in order to share the rewards was against themselves. What else were these nobles risking their men's lives for? For Christ? The Greeks were Christians. For chivalry? They were wheeling their horses and flaunting their colours as if it was a tournament and their ladies were watching whilst the minstrels and jongleurs sang their praises. The oldest and wisest of them was younger in the world outside romance than Kit. They would attack tomorrow and show their prowess and if they died their place in heaven would be in the choir of angels above the common lot. Chivalry has a lot to answer for.

When he returned to the camp there was consternation among the men of St. Foy. One of them had been caught thieving from the Venetians and was going to be hanged. Kit immediately thought of Bishop but then Bishop was unlikely to be caught. Gentleman and Soldier were dead, Lawyer had turned legitimate, Deuce might be anywhere, Bishop, no, it must be ...

He ran with the others to the banks of the Golden Horn. The Doge's galley had been rowed across to show the crusaders Venetian justice. The Doge was in his chair surrounded by his captains who were looking up to the mast-head where, at his signal, a man with a rope round his neck would be pushed off by two sailors. Kit knew it was Poet before he saw him. He was small and pale and his long fair hair was lifted by the breeze and caught by the sun. The crusaders on the bank started shouting at the Venetians, impugning their ancestry and making unholy gestures with their fingers. Kit called on them to be quiet as Poet was speaking. His voice came clear across the water.

"When you talk of me say I had good intentions but bad habits. Say that I took the Cross for Jesus and not for that drunken debauch they call Alexius emperor of Byzantium. Say that a rogue like me, a rhymer, dared to find a rhyme for Constantinople - God bless the hopeful. Say that the man who came to this noble vessel to ask to be the first warrior to cross the flying bridge, to give his life for Christ, now gives it for folly, for a little gold piece that asked to be taken from the gentleman's coat. The man who came to cross the bridge of glory must now cross the bridge of sighs. Send my tattered coat home to Ireland to my blind old Uncle Flyn, as old and blind as your famous Doge of Venice, queen of cities. Sure I took the piece for blind old Uncle Flyn to save him from starvation. I see you are impatient for justice. I thank God I was caught so my soul might be saved and go instead of me to the Holy City of God, which I would have saved single-handed if I could."

If Kit was moved who knew him, so were the Venetians who did not. The Doge turned to one of his attendants who ran to the mast and called to the sailors to release Poet, who climbed down and flung himself at the Doge's feet. Dandolo put out a hand to touch his head.

"How old is this Flyn?" he asked.

"Older than the hills, your honour."

"You will not live as long as him. Go."

Walking back to the camp Poet appeared less affected by his ordeal than Kit.

"The old boy knew I was guilty but his people wouldn't have liked it. They're all thieves anyway."

"Why?" asked Kit.

"We're all cursed with desire for one thing or another. It's a religion, an organ played by God. 'I'll give you what you want,' he says, 'next time.' Do you think there is a next time Kit?"

"I know there is." The blood was caked on his thigh.

"You must be a saint or an idiot. Take what you want this time or you'll never get it. Don't you think that's what they're after? Your old blind man, he's worse than Uncle Flyn."

Poet looked back at the sprawling city behind them.

"They promised," said Kit, "they promised we'd go to the Holy Land."

Poet sighed. "Never change Kit, never change."

Back in the camp the Squire was pacing about waiting for Kit. "Where have you been? My lord wants Thunderer ready first thing tomorrow. We're going to attack!"

In the night when God is nearer and the soul wakes up, Kit decided to tell Aimery about the miracle. It was too important to be kept secret. If Kit was destined to go to Jerusalem so was the crusade. It would ensure success against the walls of the city. He slept so peacefully after this that it must have been true.

The fourth day was woken up by drums and trumpets calling the crusaders to arms. Kit was awake before that, eagerly waiting to go to Aimery. He ran to Aimery's pavilion and, thinking a message from God was more urgent than a priest's devotions, pulled aside the curtains and went in.

There was a naked woman lying on the bed and a naked Aimery advancing and proceeding to perform an act that was as absurd as it was disturbing. Kit reeled back in a confusion of incredulity and humiliation. As children can feel the shame of their parents he felt a dishonour Aimery never felt. He hurried back to Thunderer and put his head against his flank and felt a true heart beating.

All around the camp was being broken, tents struck and baggage loaded on the wagons. In an increasing anger at the world, Kit threw on Thunderer's armour and put on his page's tabard blazoned with the black falcon. Robert's sword was leaning against the wall and he took it and went outside and looked at the walls of the city shining in the sun like an impenetrable ring of fire. He was now a page and expected to fight beside his lord. He decided to die in the siege. The blood meant not that he was going to Jerusalem but that he was going to Christ.

Lord Robert was sent with a message to the Doge that the crusaders were going to cross the Golden Horn and set up camp opposite to the wall where it turned to cross the peninsula to the sea of Marmara. Robert rode Thunderer and Kit was on the Sergeant's horse and carrying the crusader's banner. They covered a mile before reaching the Venetian ships. A skiff took them to the Doge's galley. All around them the sailors were preparing for war. The Doge listened as Robert read out the message and the old man waved his hand to show the activity in his ships.

"We also will attack the walls, my lord, but here where we can get close to them."

Robert grimaced at the old fool's stupidity. Kit thought it was lucky he was blind. Robert spoke.

"We'll be miles apart."

"So will they," said the Doge.

Robert swore most of the way back. Kit was silent, overwhelmed by the prospect of a glorious death.

The army had assembled in its divisions. The baggage train and the wagons carrying the timbers and beams to be assembled into siege engines were all beflagged and bannered in bright colours that belied the blind stupidity of the venture. It seemed as if Kit's wish would be granted.

It took most of the day for the march up the inlet to the bridge which could only be crossed by a few men at a time. Then they marched back until the walls of the city loomed some fifty feet above them and made camp on rising ground, the tents crowded within a palisade. Kit left Thunderer with the other horses in a stockade and went to observe the scene of his coming martyrdom.

He was at the corner of the city where the walls along the Golden Horn and those that stretched away three miles to the sea of Marmara met at a place called Blachernae after the imperial palace behind them. They were built of huge blocks of stone and were interspersed with towers. They had kept invaders out of Constantinople for almost a thousand years. Kit was struck by their immensity. The domes of the Blachernae palace topped the walls and it seemed as if everything in this city was bigger than anywhere else.

"Big isn't it?" Deuce was standing behind him.

"I don't know the word for it."

"Cyclopean."

"Yes," said Kit, wondering what that was.

"Wonder of the world," said Deuce, "you could go at them for fifty years and you'd never get in."

"We will."

"How do you know?"

Once more Kit was silent and once more Deuce said, "You don't, do you?" and he added, "They say the Virgin Mary protects them."

And Kit added silently, "Christ expects me."

It took six days for the Generals to prepare the assault, six days during which the crusaders were under attack by bowmen on the parapets and raids by skirmishers from the city. Kit was sent backwards and forwards through the camp with orders from the Generals to Lord Robert and from him to whoever he could think of. He passed men making scaling ladders, others dragging the stone-throwing engines from place to place, more skulking and skiving to avoid doing anything. All of them were subdued by the shadow of the walls. The priests moved amongst them, assuring them that the Greeks were worse than Saracens because they called themselves Christians but were preventing the crusade from sailing to the Holy Land. What was preventing them was the lack of money.

They went to war, drums and trumpets, the lords on their chargers, the sword-bearers Kit amongst them, even the common men wearing their crosses as if they were going to a tourney. The main force halted a few hundred yards from the walls whilst Hugh of St. Blois led his division forward under a spattering of bolts and arrows to within bow-shot. A body of almost a hundred men carrying a long battering-ram ran ahead. Kit thought of a house he had once built of sand and knocked down with a stick. They reached the base of the wall, the ram swung, struck, shuddered, the men were flung aside under a deadly avalanche of rocks from the parapet. The squads of ladder-men followed, twenty or so and raised the scaling-ladders for the chosen heroes to climb. Few reached the parapet and they were knocked down with pikes and poles and fell like discarded toys broken and disjointed, only toys do not scream. Those who followed had no option but to climb on to receive the same casual fate. Over his head Kit saw rocks and boulders flung from a mangonel or trebuchet fly over the wall or crash harmlessly into it. Incredibly, the lords let it go on because they did not know what else to do. The heaps of bodies rose to the fourth and fifth rungs of the ladders. The cries mingled with the shouts of triumph from the wall. Still they climbed. A sergeant and a few men gained a narrow foothold, a forlorn hope ended by a Varangian axe. Was this the death Kit wanted? Hugh of Blois turned his horse and rode back through the ranks, the signal to retreat. The crusaders turned and walked back in silence. There was no silence at the foot of the wall for some time.

A message came from the Doge of Venice. Kit was there when it was read aloud to the officers. The currents in the sea had prevented the ships from closing with the walls. He had ordered his men to disembark onto the narrow strip of land below them and had led the landing himself. There were few defenders there, mostly militia and the Venetians had breached a gate and entered the city. He could not advance without more men. He begged the Generals to send him a division to take advantage of the success he had gained.

The Generals shook their heads. They were about to repeat the disaster and resume the assault. They were saved from further disgrace by the drums beating an alarm call from the camp and a white-faced messenger riding up to Hugh. The order was given to return to the camp with all haste. Hugh spoke to Robert who dismounted and gave Thunderer's reins to Kit.

"Go to the Venetians! Demand to see the Doge. They will know you by my colours. A great army is coming from the city to attack us! He must come at once. Repeat it!"

Kit did and mounted Thunderer.

"Ride! Our lives depend on it!"

Kit rode past the ladders standing like grave markers in heaps of death and on the route he had taken before with Robert. As the Venetian ships came in sight he was amazed. The wind had changed and driven the five huge transports against the wall. The flying bridges were secured to the parapet and the towers as far as he could see were flying the flag of Venice's patron saint St. Mark. The Doge and his officers were still on the strip of land. The rowers from the galleys were coming ashore well-armed and entering a broken gate in the wall. Kit jumped off Thunderer and ran towards the Doge's chair. He was recognised by the guard and led before Dandolo.

"You have come to tell me the Generals are sending me a division," said the Doge.

Kit repeated his message. He was made to repeat it again. The Doge turned his head away as if his blind eyes had seen something he disliked.

"They demand? I must come at once? I have an open door to the city. Tell them to come here." Kit's heart missed a beat. "No, no, they cannot tell Venice what to do." Kit had failed. The crusade was over. Kit knelt and touched the Doge's feet. He looked up like a child and in a child's voice spoke.

"For Christ's sake my lord, save us."

At that moment only a child could have reached out and touched the old man's heart. The officers and captains standing by, proud men, felt an instinctive resolve to respond to the cry of a child.

The Doge raised his hand and touched Kit's head.

"I see your face," he said.

He was giving up his victory for Kit.

The orders were shouted from man to man, the trumpets sounded and amid the consternation it caused the Venetians began to retreat to their ships.

Kit rose to his feet, he could not wait. He bowed as deeply as he could and turned and ran back to where Thunderer was being held by a guard. As he rode he turned and looked back and saw smoke rising from the part of the city occupied by the Venetians. They had set fire to the houses to cover their retreat.

The crusaders' camp was deserted. Kit rode on and came across Montferrat's division standing as the rearguard. He saw the cooks and grooms had been called up to protect the camp, a strange company wearing quilts and horse blankets, helmets made out of cooking-pots and basins and armed with pitchforks, knives and pestles. Rounding the angle of the walls where the Blachernae palace stood, he glanced up and saw Byzantine ladies and their maids watching from the windows. He rode into the sunlight on the plain and the ranks of the crusader army, thin enough, perhaps three thousand foot and five hundred horse, drawn up in three divisions. He reined in Thunderer and trotted to the front. Louis of Blois, Baldwin of Flanders, Hugh of St. Pol, were sitting like statues at the head of the mounted lords, squires and sergeants. Lord Robert turned his horse to meet him.

"Are they coming?"

"Yes my lord."

"They'll be too late."

Leaving Thunderer to blow, Robert went to report to his lord Louis of Blois. Before he dismounted Kit looked across the plain. It was mid-afternoon and the sun was in his eyes. He raised his hand to shade them and the haze in the distance resolved into a vast army, the Sergeant said thirty thousand, covering the ground and slowly moving towards them. He had no thought of death. Robert returned and they changed horses. Kit took Robert's sword from the Squire.

"Don't drop it." The Squire had never liked him.

They waited knowing they would have to charge because there was no defence. As the enemy approached, these Christians were the enemy, Kit could distinguish the mercenaries on both flanks from the Greeks in the centre. The Varangian Guards were escorting a group of priests carrying crosses and icons and a man in purple who Kit thought must be the Emperor. If this was for Christ, which side was Christ on? He was shaken out of his wonder by the order "Spur!"

The lords took their lances from the squires and spurred their horses to walk on. Behind them the foot-soldiers picked up their weapons and followed them.

Between the two armies the ground rose slightly where a canal bed had been cut that brought water to the city. The crusaders reached the top of the rise and halted. The front ranks of the Byzantines appeared almost within bow-shot and the archers and bowmen on both sides exchanged futile arrows. The impasse could have lasted the rest of the day but Baldwin's charger moved forward, Kit never knew if it was from the master's or the horse's impatience. Someone shouted "Trot!" and the Flanders division set off down the long slope to the canal. Hugh and Louis were not to be outdone and spurred on their divisions. Kit was riding behind Robert and he felt the terrible attraction of a challenge to his bravery that leads a man on to death. Then he saw they were passing Baldwin's line and they were heading for the canal. They were now within bow-shot and the lords raised their shields and perhaps their doubts, because if they managed to cross the canal they would have to charge up the slope the other side where the enemy would have the advantage.

They did not charge, nor did the Emperor's army advance further than the bank on their side. Perhaps someone had seen the masts of the Venetian ships in the Golden Horn? Perhaps the Emperor had achieved his aim to make the Venetians withdraw from the city? The crusaders stood and watched as the Byzantine army melted away like snow in summer.

The return to camp was more a funeral procession than a triumphal march. In camp the flags drooped, so did the men and dragged their feet and made no noise. They had been defeated at the wall and lost many comrades, the Venetians had been deprived of their victory and the Emperor's army was unscathed. Tiredness and shortage of provisions depressed their bodies and the failure of the crusade their spirits. Summer was hot, the acrid smell of burning was in the air and fumes stung their nostrils. Over all drifted the black cupola of smoke from the crucible of Constantinople, as Poet put it.

"It's better than being dead," said Kit.

"God bless the hopeful," said Poet quoting himself.

They were outside Lord Robert's pavilion and Kit was polishing his armour.

"Did you not know that when you're dead you can go wherever you like? If in your life you were bound for Jerusalem you'll go to Jerusalem and if you were bound for Tipperary you'll go to Tipperary, even though it's further than Jerusalem?"

"What the preacher said in chapel is true?"

"If you believe it, Kit. The trouble is did he believe it, or like the rest of the priesthood did he say it without understanding what he was saying?"

Kit looked puzzled.

"When you were a child and your mam told you stories that were made up by Uncle Flyn himself did she believe them true?"

"I didn't have a mam," said Kit and it was the first time he had told himself.

"I knew you were one of the little people."

Poet did not say more and Kit was offended. He saw Deuce coming out of the Marquis of Montferrat's pavilion, not by the back door where they emptied the slops but under the embroidered awning at the front - and attended by Montferrat the leader of the crusade. Kit shook Poet's arm and they watched as Montferrat patted Deuce's shoulder and gave him a flask stamped with his own cipher. Deuce came their way jauntily.

"Come with me!"

He led them to the usual place by the Golden Horn where the city filled their vision, marred by the evil smoke covering it.

"It's ours," said Deuce.

"Hours to what?" asked Poet, "Another attack?"

"Ours! Ours! Belonging to us! The Emperor's gone boys, did a flit before somebody did it for him."

Deuce took a swig from the flask and passed it to Poet.

"Nectar of the gods," said Poet and passed it to Kit.

Kit shook his shoulders as if he knew what to expect and then got what he did not, his first taste of good wine - revolting!

"Lovely," he said.

Deuce was jubilant.

"Kit my boy, you were right all the time. You said we'd go to the Holy Land. You said we'd take Constantinople. I knew you knew something."

"Did he go just like that?" asked Poet.

"It was the shame of the retreat, thirty to one! They were watching from the windows to see us slaughtered. Then it was the fire, a third of the city's gone up in smoke. Nobody liked him."

"What next?"

"They've gone to sober up Alexius."

Kit looked up. Alexius would be emperor and pay them what he had promised and they would go to the Holy Land at last. O God, O thank God. He took another swig to prove he was a man and got sick.

Later he saw Alexius being carried to the pavilion and wondered why men drank.

A delegation of great men dressed with barbaric splendour came from the city and were escorted to the pavilion. The Generals had assembled and Kit was in his tabard with the pages forming a guard of honour. The page nearest the entrance heard what was going on and passed the word along the line. They had come for Alexius but not to make him emperor. His father, old blind Isaac, had been freed from jail and put on the throne. Montferrat was protesting he could not trust them and they could not have Alexius until Isaac agreed to the terms negotiated at Zara. The pages stood to attention as the delegation swept out disappointed, they had the king they wanted but not the pawn.

"As long as we've got him," said the smart one, "we've got them."

"Why?" asked Kit, but nobody bothered to answer. The army was ordered to stand to.

The next day the Generals sent their own delegation into the city. They returned in triumph with a treaty signed and sealed by the new Emperor confirming every detail of the one made with Alexius - 200,000 silver marks, provisions for a year, 10,000 soldiers to join the crusade and the Greek church placed under the authority of Pope Innocent. Kit recalled the day in the long grass with Alexius.

One of the pages had gone with the delegation and the others eagerly surrounded him to hear his story.

It was a fairy tale but true. The Blachernae palace was a treasure-house. The halls were marble with mosaics dotted with real gold pieces. The Varangian Guards Kit had fought in the tower wore magnificent uniforms, the courtiers more magnificent and the ladies ... the page was breathless. The Emperor, a little old man in purple and jewels, perched on a golden throne under a golden crown, like a … the boy paused … the puppet Herod in the travelling miracle play, except his strings were pulled by the great men behind the throne. The Empress … the page's lord came out and Kit never knew.

Now the Generals had the treaty they no longer needed Alexius and he was escorted into Constantinople with all the pomp he could have desired. There was still a deep distrust of the Greeks and the army was ordered to break camp and return to Galata on the far side of the Golden Horn. Unwisely, the crusaders were allowed to visit the city when they were off duty. It was like inviting children into a sweetshop with their hands tied.

The smart young page who had made a point of displaying his superiority to Kit now decided to adopt him as a disciple. They had more time to spend together as their lords were pursuing their pleasures in the city. His name was Qenet Alaric de Clairon, which overawed Kit as much as his composure and urbanity. He allowed Kit to call him Alaric. He planned a trip into Constantinople. "It's not Paris but it has a gross attraction rather like an elephant."

On a day in July when the sun was high and the sky was blue a boatman rowed them across the Golden Horn. They entered the city through the gate broken open by the Venetians. All this area had suffered from the fire and they walked between burnt and blackened houses for almost an hour before they came to the wide street that had stopped the blaze and led them into the centre of the city. Five domes of a church shone over the rooftops like five rising suns. It was the church of the twelve apostles and the old Greek guide told them that seven of them lay inside. Mosaics flecked with gold covered the walls with scenes from the life of Christ. They saw a mausoleum where umpteen early emperors were buried under marble and gold leaf as if there had been an earthquake in a quarry. The old man looked round cautiously and said they could see something few had seen, but for a drachma. Alaric nodded and he led them to a chancel where there was nothing but the stump of a broken column.

"There," said the old man, "That's where He was scourged."

It was a moment before Kit's heart lurched. "He" was Christ. Alaric pulled him away and hurried him out before the guide got his drachma.

Along the street the houses grew bigger and more elaborate. The street became a colonnade between stalls and shops full of goods St.

Foy had never seen. A Roman aqueduct carried water from the canal and a pink marble column soared into the sky remembering some emperor or other.

They turned into a triumphal way as broad as six chariots that led into a square that could have swallowed Paris. There was a victory column that cricked Kit's neck and an emperor on a horse treading on a wretched captive.

"That's you," said Alaric.

Another square, this time for Constantine himself surrounded by his plunder, fantastic bronze Greek statues of the gods and goddesses, Athene, Hera, Aphrodite, three times life-size. Alaric lingered.

They turned towards the sea and on the far side of yet another square saw St. Sophia under the sun against a blue sky. The dome was even more impressive from inside, unsupported and so high that Christ in a mosaic covering the whole surface looked no bigger than a man. Windows around the base illuminated the coloured marble pillars and mosaics on the walls like an illustrated missal. The altar-table was overlaid with gold and glittering crushed jewels and stood under a silver canopy supported by silver columns. Everywhere Kit looked there was a treasure reflecting the glory of - what, he wondered? Christ? Wealth? Power? Then he saw the simple stone cover of the well on which Christ had sat when he talked to the Samaritan woman and his wonder dwindled to the answer - the glory of man.

Alaric was becoming impatient. There were more statues outside in a square, a huge clock, a giant weather-vane, a triumphal arch, a bronze gate, a vast arena for racing chariots and over the entrance four enormous copper horses in full gallop. Another statue.

"Alaric, what's that?"

"An elephant. Come on."

"We haven't seen the Great Palace."

"We can't somebody lives there."

Alaric dragged him back to the business quarter behind the docks along the Bosporus. There the streets were full of men with a purpose, merchants, money-lenders, stall-holders, clerks, priests, buyers and sellers of every nationality. Constantinople was the jewelled ring on the finger of Europe that almost touched the cheek of Asia, as Poet said later.

They entered a street of taverns and houses that nobody lived in. Men were hurrying up and down the steps with fixed expressions. Nobody seemed to recognise anybody else. This was where Alaric wanted to be and he pulled Kit up the steps of a house and through the doorway.

The windows of the room were curtained and it was a moment before Kit could see. There were plush cushioned alcoves with small tables with candles on them and drapes behind. A single man sat in each alcove being served with wine by a series of young women. When the man finished his drink he turned the glass upside down and went out with the woman who had brought it through the drapes. Alaric pushed him into an alcove and sat and waited.

"I've given up drinking," said Kit.

A woman came with a flask of viscous yellow wine and two glasses. She looked askance at Kit, shrugged her shoulders and left. Another woman came and filled the glasses. Alaric drank half of his and pointed at Kit to make him drink. It was foul and burnt his throat. A third woman came, younger than the others and Alaric swallowed the rest and turned the glass upside down. The woman came round the table, took Alaric's arm and led him off through the drapes. "Wait for me," he told Kit.

Kit reddened. It was Aimery again. He jumped up and ran outside to wait in the street. Barely three minutes later Alaric came out white-faced and shaking.

"What happened?" asked Kit.

"I changed my mind," said Alaric, "nothing happened."

Kit thought it was probably the other way round. Nothing had happened and then Alaric had changed his mind. But he did not say so. They walked back to the gate in silence.

Kit settled into the routine life of a soldier in camp. He rode out on Thunderer nearly every morning and saw to his needs before his own and then Lord Robert's. He had time to reflect on his experiences and his destiny. The first had taken him from a solitary life of drudgery to one of the company of men and horses, heraldic glamour and the terrible excitement of war. At the age of thirteen or fourteen he did not know, he thought he had become a man. The second destiny was the one he had foreseen in the chapel at St. Foy, Jerusalem. There was a forest of ifs to go through, if Alexius kept his promise, if the Generals kept theirs made at Corfu to quit Constantinople in a month, if the debt to the Venetians was paid, if … he came out into the clearing of his vision of the Holy City. One if was felled when Robert announced he was going to attend the coronation of Alexius as co-emperor with his father on the first of August 1203. Old Isaac was a broken puppet and the great men needed another.

Alexius's first act was to pay 100,000 silver marks, half of what he had promised to the crusaders. He needed them to stay to protect him from his own people and his uncle who was still considered to be emperor by the greater part of the Byzantine empire. Half of the money went to the Venetians whose deal with the crusaders ended in September, but what happened to the rest?

"The nobs got it," said Deuce.

He had been in the city where there was an increasing resentment against the payment which had been raised by sequestering the property of the ex-emperor's supporters and impounding the gold and silver ornaments of the churches.

They were sitting staring at the city.

"There's a lot of ifs," said Kit, "and only one but."

"What's that?"

"Christ."

Disillusion came with the night. It was not dark but sticky. He woke to see blood on his thighs and this time the source was obvious. It could not be another miracle. It had to be natural. He was glad he was not a woman.

In one way it was a relief. Divine intervention could work both ways, if God can read our thoughts we must think again. If it was nature he could not help it. Unless God was nature, or nature God. Too many thoughts he thought and slept with the ease of a child. An old man would have thought all night long and still not have thought of an answer.

The new Emperor came to visit his old friends. The council was held in the Doge's pavilion. Deuce had found the privy occupied and was sitting outside with Kit and Poet.

"The nobs would leave here if they could. Alexius is terrified and will offer them anything to stay. And old Dandolo you never know, he sees a lot for a blind man."

"What rhymes with Venice?" asked Poet.

"We're going to Jerusalem," said Kit.

"Have you been talking to the fairies again?"

"If we don't go soon," said Deuce, "it will be too late. The Venetians will be off in September."

"You can't stop a crusade." Kit was adamant.

"No," said Poet, "but you can turn it around."

The council was breaking up and they sprang to attention. Kit fetched Thunderer. Lord Robert was talking to Count Louis.

"What did Alexius mean, take us into his service?"

"To keep us here Robert, to keep us waiting for the rest of our money as a threat to his disloyal subjects. He promises to provision the army and renew our lease of the Venetian ships for another year and he swore we'd be in the Holy Land by March next year."

"Do you believe him, my lord?"

"Of course not. But what's the alternative? To go now with no money, to end up in some garrison city on the coast of the Holy Land for winter?"

"To keep our word to God."

"Don't you dare accuse me of being forsworn! It's the only way."

Louis marched off to join the Generals in an awkward meeting with the crusaders to explain why they could not keep their word.

"Watch out for people who say it's the only way," said Poet, "it means no exit."

There was trouble in the city and the crusaders were confined to camp. Kit laughed, now Alaric would never find out if he could.

In spite of their confinement stories circulated of the incredible folly of Alexius. Kit had witnessed his charm, his indiscretion and his vindictiveness. In the two weeks after his coronation he managed to outrage the great families of Constantinople by extortion, the church by robbery, the citizens by drinking and cavorting openly with young crusader aides-de-camp and the mob by failing to reward them for ousting his uncle and for keeping the hated crusaders who had attacked them across the Golden Horn as a threat. He particularly annoyed the Patriarch of the Greek Church by commanding him to write to Pope Innocent agreeing to his subjection to Rome. The venerable old man replied that the only thing Rome ever did for Christ was to crucify Him.

At this critical moment, in his vanity Alexius decided to lead a campaign to capture his uncle and subdue the provinces that still acknowledged him as emperor. Montferrat joined the venture having been bribed with Greek gold and his division was not averse to the opportunity of pillaging the neighbourhood. Alexius's best chance to maintain his authority marched out of the city at the end of the second week.

Within days a Greek mob entered the Latin quarter to loot and burn churches, warehouses, dockyards and the residences of the traders and merchants who had lived there for many years. Many of those took to their ships and sailed to the Golden Horn to join the crusader camp.

The next night, a band of raiders rowed across from the camp and attacked an isolated mosque outside the walls to cover others who infiltrated the city and set fires in the nearest buildings. Lord Robert's company was put on alert and he rode with the Sergeant, Kit and an escort to the tower of Galata. Kit was sent up to the roof to report.

It was a warm night and he could see more stars than he ever believed possible. The water below the tower was darker than the sky. Where they flowed into the Bosporus small waves stirred by the wind reflected the stars. A spark of light drew his eyes to the city. The mosque was somewhere in the darkness below the walls but above them was a red aura rising with the smoke in which it was reflected. Kit called down, "There's fires inside the walls." As he watched, flickering spires of flame shot up from many places and there was the faint murmur of a fire. "They're getting bigger."

In what seemed seconds the smoke flared red and yellow and the towers were black against the bale fire. The wind surged as if sucked in by a furnace.

"Flames, flames!" cried Kit.

"Come down," said the Sergeant, "we can see them."

"There's a boat!"

A fishing boat with ten or twelve rowers was heading for the mooring under the tower where the great chain had been.

"They're coming ashore!"

"I've got them," said the Sergeant.

Now the flames were leaping higher than the walls and the murmur became a roar and the smoke was red and rising in the wind. Kit thought he heard screams or the cries of gulls. He hoped they were the cries of gulls.

He ran down to where the boat had scraped against the base of the tower and the rowers and some twenty men were lined up against a wall guarded by the company. Robert rode up on Thunderer.

"Sergeant, do you know these men?"

"Some of them, my lord."

"And the others?"

"They look like civilians."

"Hold the ones you recognise and let the others go."

Robert rode back to camp.

The Sergeant took Kit along the line and held up a lantern to look at their faces. Those he passed by slipped away into the darkness. Those he stopped were seized by the crusaders.

Kit had already seen the fat man halfway down the line. He was a thief and a murderer. He was also a companion who had taken Kit into his company. He was only two men away.

The Sergeant stopped and looked at the fat man carefully, raising the lantern to see the black-grimed face. Then he tapped the fat man's jerkin and it clinked.

Kit was watching and he saw the fat man's hand move towards his belt where Kit knew he had a knife. He stepped between the fat man and the Sergeant.

"I know him sir. He's all right."

Soldiers have a code more compelling than the code of law, a comradeship established by endurance and confidence in each other. The Sergeant recognised it and though he knew the boy was lying he moved on to the next man. Bishop slipped away without a word.

The crusaders watched the fire spreading over the city for six or seven days, seeming to die down and then flaring up in another place like a horrible plague on a dying man. There was a fascination and a dread, a fear for their fellow creatures being burnt alive, or if they escaped the flames losing their livelihoods in them. Those who had fled from the city were horrified as the smoke rose over places they knew - "Look, it's coming from the market place!" "Oh God save us, Saint Sophia!" "The pillar of Constantine!" They blamed Alexius but they knew the criminals were crusaders. Later when they were able to return to their homes they could not find them and though the great cathedral had been spared, many dead saints and emperors were now nameless heaps of dust and ashes. In the meantime Alexius was campaigning in Thrace.

But what of Kit? Bishop had left a gold platen under the straw in Thunderer's stable. He wished Bishop had robbed him instead of loading him with shame, guilt and the dread of being discovered. He was desperate to get rid of it as soon as he could and thought of Poet who always needed money.

"I knew you were a thief, Kit."

"It wasn't me. Bishop gave it me."

"Then you must keep it or he'll be insulted. He's a devil of a man and if he saw me with it he'd say I stole it from you. Don't you know that a thief thinks all men are thieves and related to Uncle Flyn? That's how he justifies his thievery. It's the same with all rogues and murderers. Just as the priest tells us we're all good at heart and tortures us to get the goodness out of us. A great lord you might think fears nothing, can't sleep at night because he's terrified we're all lords-in-waiting and will murder him in his bed for his title and his lands. Sure, isn't that the way his ancestors got them?"

Kit did not doubt it and Poet went on.

"Did you see the columns and the statues of the emperors glorifying them for what, Kit? For killing their brothers and uncles who would have killed them. Did you see the grand stone pictures of the saints? What did they do? They got themselves killed because they thought that was what God wanted. Doesn't God kill us all in the end and they thought they'd get it in first. There only ever was one good man and his wife fixed it for him with an apple."

"I thought you were going to say Christ."

"Him we're here for, Kit? Or is it for ourselves, our souls, our making up for our sins? If it is then every man's his own Christ and Christ is all men."

"Poet, what shall I do with the plate?"

"Give the horse his feed on it."

Kit sat and thought for a long time until Thunderer wondered if he was ever going to get his dinner. Eventually Kit decided to find Deuce.

The best way to find Deuce was to let him find you, so Kit went into Lord Robert's pavilion and came out looking furtive. He heard the hiss as he passed the cook-shop.

"Kit it's me. What do you know?"

"I know where to find a gold plate."

"I'll come with you!"

They walked back to the stable and Kit fed Thunderer.

"Where is it?"

"Under the straw."

Deuce found the platen and examined it.

"It's real gold. You never know with the church. Whose is it?"

Kit did not want to mention Bishop.

"I suppose it's mine."

Deuce put it back under the straw.

"Good luck to you."

"Don't you want it?"

"Not if it was the last one in the world. It's yours and we're brothers. I'd never take it from you."

"I'm giving it to you."

"No Kit, what we steal we keep. Otherwise there would be bad blood between us. If you wanted it later you'd hate me for having it."

Deuce left and Kit was in despair until he thought of Alaric.

Alaric was a gentleman and would take anything from anybody.

He told Alaric he had found it and that it was too good for him to keep.

"That's decent of you, Kit. I can't remember where I lost it."

Kit rather hoped it would be discovered in Alaric's possession but nobody ever searches a gentleman.

It was autumn and the sun dipped lower in the sky, tinting pink the wisps of smoke still rising from the city. The crusaders in the camp had little to do but wait for Alexius and Montferrat to return. They heard through spies and informers that the people were turning against the two emperors, not so much the poor who were told to blame the crusaders, but those who had the most to gain from a revolution, as always, those in the middle who wanted to be on top. Old Isaac was demented they said and young Alexius was not there. They looked around for another puppet and by mistake chose a man bolder and more devious than they were themselves.

In Montferrat's absence the Generals met in Count Louis' pavilion and Robert was there and so was Kit. The Doge had retired to his galley in the Golden Horn from where he could ponder over the crusaders and the city. Enrico Dandolo controlled the game. The crusaders could not move without his ships. The emperor, whoever he was, knew that the flying bridges on those ships could breach the walls of the city. Dandolo had only to wait to see which side offered Venice the best chance to achieve its goal, dominance of the seas and the valuable east-west trade.

The Generals were talking.

"This new man, what's his name?" asked Louis.

"Mouro ... Mouzo ... Moo ... I don't know, it ends in opholus," said Robert.

"They all do. How do you spell it?"

"I can't even pronounce it. The spy said he wears green slippers."

"That doesn't mean anything."

"It means a great deal in Constantinople. He's related to one of the old emperors."

"The place is full of them! The real rulers are behind the throne. What are we to do, Robert?"

"My lord?"

"The men think we betrayed them by bringing them here. They've no money, they can't go into the city, they've got nothing to do. There's nothing more dangerous than an idle man."

Kit thought an active Saracen might be, but would they ever see one?

"My lord, we must wait for Montferrat and the Emperor," said Robert, "Alexius is an idiot and Montferrat is trying to carve himself a kingdom in Thrace or Thessaly. There are six months before we can sail for the Holy Land."

This was the one and only mention of the purpose of the crusade.

Kit was not idle but Alaric was and challenged him to a race between Thunderer and his own horse Mercury. Kit accepted providing they raced in the morning early. The course was along the banks of the Golden Horn to where it joined the river running from the foothills of a range of mountains. It was about three miles and would take less than an hour.

Early autumn and the sun was just rising when they started at an easy pace following their shadows. They watched each other and when one began to trot the other spurred his horse into a canter which became a gallop and then they were racing past the stopping point across the plain towards the hills.

Kit shouted, "Stop! Stop! I must go back!"

"Then you've lost!" cried Alaric and urged Mercury on.

"Charge!" screamed Kit and Thunderer charged past Mercury.

Alaric drew out his whip.

They chased and raced until the ground began to rise and both horses were blown and dropped to a walk. They agreed to a draw. They had been riding for two hours.

The sun was up and they were crossing slopes of tall grasses and flowers dotted with wild olive trees. Kit knew Lord Robert would be shouting and ungenerously decided to put the blame on Thunderer.

"He bolted, my lord. I couldn't stop him."

Alaric did not care.

The grass grew sparser and the ground was strewn with rocks. The mountains were nearer as if they had moved and the two boys were in a land that had not felt a footstep in a thousand years. Now they were riding past huge boulders and jagged fissures in the rock. The sun was directly overhead and they could not see their shadows. They let their reins drop and their horses find the way.

They came up on a high ridge. Below them they saw a grove of pointed trees unlike any others they had seen and a bright blue mountain pool. The horses scented water. They wound their way down and dismounted to let them drink.

"Where are we, Alaric?"

"Ancient Greece."

"Who lived here?"

"Ancient Greeks." Alaric took off his clothes. "I'm going to swim."

Kit did not want to look and looked. Alaric's body was young and slender like a child's, he walked like a child, he cared for nothing but the moment like a child. Kit's body was changing and hidden by his tabard or leather apron.

"Are you coming in?"

Kit shook his head. In the water Alaric was half boy and half fish as the ripples turned his skin to scales. Kit saw askance something that made him look again. There was a white figure half-hidden by the trees. Someone was watching them!

"Alaric! Someone's watching us!"

Alaric waved his hand dismissively. It was the gesture of a class beyond reproach - *sans peur et sans reproche.*

Kit went to look, he was frightened and a prey to shame.

It was dark under the trees and he picked his way round behind the white figure. He drew his page's dagger and rushed out shouting, "Die!"

He stopped dead. He was in a clearing, threatening the back of a naked woman, a white marble naked woman, a goddess with white stone ringlets, a classic face and elegant body.

Alaric appeared still naked on the far side of the clearing and stared in open-mouthed admiration.

"I wish she was real."

"She is real," said Kit, "too real."

"Let's see if there's any more." Alaric started out.

"Put some clothes on first."

"Why? They can't see us."

Kit thought they might.

They searched and found a marble god without a head and an ugly marble satyr with horns and the legs of a goat.

"It's a sacred grove if you want to … fertility."

"How do you fertility?" asked Kit, curious.

"Sexual stuff. You know." Kit blushed. "You look like a girl."

"It's supposed to be a crusade," said Kit.

"I'm going back to the pool." Alaric disappeared in the trees.

The headless god had only lost his head, everything else was fully exposed including his penis. Kit thought, Christ was a man and in the statues, mosaics, the rood screen, Christ was always covered. Why? Was God ashamed of His creation? Was the church ashamed of God? Was it prudish? Kit knew about prudes, the old nuns in the priory were prudes and had made him wear an undergarment because his skirt rode up when he was kneeling to scrub the floor. He remembered his oath, the crusader's oath to go in arms to the Holy Sepulchre in Jerusalem. He was in a sacred grove in Ancient Greece looking at an ancient Greek god with a penis. Was the shame to him or to the great lords who had twisted his mission? What did Christ want with Jerusalem? He had been betrayed there, condemned there, whipped and crucified there. Why did Kit the waif, the drudge, want to go there?

Alaric was shouting, "We've got to go back!"

Go back? He had never been there. Then it came to him, he had to go there so that he could go back, as Christ in death went back. It was a pilgrimage to himself, so that one day he could return, the day he died and be with Christ.

As they were riding back he turned to Alaric.

"I know why we're going on crusade."

"So do I. What else can a gentleman do?"

Kit thought he might try scrubbing the floor.

Montferrat brought Alexius and the army back to Constantinople in November, three months after they had marched away. The new emperor discovered that his empire had shrunk to the environs of the city and even that was on the verge of revolt. The resentment of the Greeks against the crusaders, who they called barbarians, had festered into a great boil of hatred. Old Isaac had drifted into the fog of senility with visions of himself being raised to heaven having been murdered by his ungrateful son.

The crusaders had their own hatred of the Greeks who they believed had cheated them. Alexius still owed them 100,000 marks and they were no nearer the Holy Land than they were when they arrived. Now they could not leave until March the following year, when the Venetian ships could sail without the peril of capsizing or being flung against a rocky coast. All soldiers complain but they had good reason, two years from home and a doubtful outcome.

Lord Robert shouted more than ever and his bad temper went down the line of command until it reached Kit at the bottom.

"It's that god-forsaken idiot Alexius!"

Count Louis was concerned.

"Keep your voice down Robert, there could be spies around."

There were.

Deuce had been inside the city.

"How do you get in and out without being discovered?" asked Kit.

"That's my secret," said Deuce.

Poet laughed, "He borrows a donkey and a string of onions and the smell's so strong nobody wants to go near him."

"Now I won't be able to do it again!"

"Nobody's listening."

"There are spies everywhere."

They were sitting looking at the cause of all the trouble, the great sprawling city, the biggest in the world.

"As I was saying," said Deuce, "they don't like Alexius because he brought us here and as long as we're here they can't get rid of him. We don't like Alexius because he brought us here and he hasn't kept his promises. He knows we have to leave in March and so he puts off paying us. He's stuck with us, we're stuck with them and they're stuck with him."

"That's beautiful," said Poet.

"When is March?" asked Kit.

"When the flowers come out at home," said Poet.

"They're out here now."

"Yes Kit, so are we."

Having heard from Kit how Deuce fooled the Greeks and got into the city Alaric decided to do the same. The secret grove had cast its spell and he was dreaming of a white goddess and a red-plush alcove. It was dangerous, there were brawls and killings every day.

Why did Kit go with him? Just as he had protected Bishop who had befriended him, so he did Alaric. He had never had a friend in St. Foy.

They did not take a donkey but a boat. Dressed as fishermen, Alaric rubbed Kit's rough coat with a herring and bought him a basket of sardines. They paid a boatman to row them across to the city at dusk and wait for them until morning. Alaric had some Greek, he had managed to stay at his studies for a year or two and told the guards at the gate their boat had sunk and they had to be at the market in the morning. They held their noses and let them in. Alaric headed straight for the house of his dreams and Kit tagged along, an unhappy acolyte. He was left outside.

"No one's going to come near you."

He sat on the steps until he saw lanterns and heard the tapping sticks of the night-watch. He dropped the basket and dodged into the area hoping they would not smell him. They smelt the basket of fish and took it for their supper.

An hour went by and Kit began to worry. Alaric might have been drugged and robbed or stabbed for the gold chain he wore. The basement had a small window which he prised open. He had to take off the coat to squeeze inside. He was in a cellar with stairs up to a door with light coming through the cracks. He crept up and opened it and was immediately seized by two half-dressed women. He wriggled in their grasp and it became obvious to them what he was.

"It's a girl!"

They let him go.

"Poor creature, she must be hungry."

With the inborn sympathy for a hungry girl they took him to the kitchen. There was a fat man, in an apron and a starched linen cap by the stove.

"A girl broke in poor thing, she must be starving."

The fat man turned. Kit nearly cried out. It was Bishop. A cook in a brothel.

"Leave her to me, I'll fix her up."

The women left. Bishop laughed.

"You're a clever one Kit, I'd never have thought of being a girl!"

"Alaric's here! I've got to get him out!"

"Who's he?"

"My friend."

To a villain the friend of a friend is a friend until one robs the other.

"I know where he'll be."

Bishop led the way to the corridor lined with doors which Kit realised must lead to the alcoves.

"He'll be in one of these … struggle!"

Bishop grabbed his collar as a matronly woman appeared. Kit struggled.

"I've got her ma'am, the thieving little witch!"

The woman passed them.

"What's he look like?"

How could Kit describe Alaric?

"He's a nob."

"I took him his dinner. He's in here."

He opened a door. The girl on the couch was surprised.

"He hasn't done it yet."

Alaric sat up.

Bishop kept hold of Kit with one hand and got hold of Alaric with the other.

"He paid with a dud ducat!"

He dragged them both out to the corridor and back into the kitchen.

"Get out the way you came. Get back to camp quick! We're at war!"

"What about you?"

Bishop smiled. "I'm neutral."

They crawled out of the house and back to the boat. The guard at the gate was asleep.

"Who was he?" Alaric asked.

"A friend," said Kit.

They were at war.

Montferrat had returned dissatisfied. He had family connections in the Byzantine empire and high hopes for himself. He was fed up with Alexius and persuaded the Generals to send a delegation to him with an ultimatum, pay the debt or suffer the consequences. The delegation included Robert who was well in favour and at last he met Mourtzouphlus whose name he had scrambled. Alexius had unwisely taken the demagogue into his court to keep him quiet. The crusader lords were less than decorous in their approach to Alexius whom they despised. They misjudged the Byzantine temperament that prized ritual and decorum above all else. They demanded payment. Mourtzouphlus jumped up and expressed the public opinion. Robert repeated his words.

"The rascal got up and said they'd paid us too much already. 'Don't give them any more! Send them away! Make them leave the country!'" One of the more belligerent lords threatened the Emperor that if he refused they would take the money themselves. Tempers flared, hands went to knives and daggers.

The delegates hastily retreated.

The Generals went to consult the Doge. This was Dandolo's opportunity. If Alexius continued to refuse to pay, the crusaders would take the money themselves and ravage the surrounding countryside, looting and burning and he, by their original agreement, would get half the booty. If the Greeks reacted violently, it would end with an attack on the city to drive Alexius out and install a puppet emperor of their own to pay them off. He offered to mediate and arranged a meeting with Alexius in the principal harbour where he could speak from the safety of his galley. He took three galleys and Alexius rode down to the quayside to shout across the bulwarks. What he said no one in the camp knew. What was reported to have been said was spread about by the Doge's agents. Dandolo had asked Alexius to honour his word. Alexius had repeated that he would not pay any more and added that he was not afraid of the Venetians or the crusaders and he ordered the Doge to leave his harbours immediately or he would take action against him. They quoted the Doge's reply, "Wretched boy, we dragged thee out of the filth and into the filth will cast thee again!"

Kit did not believe it but the great majority of the crusaders did. War was inevitable.

The crusaders had been idle and anxious too long and were eager for action, particularly when there was little danger to themselves in sacking the churches and villas of the rich that stood outside the walls of the city. The priests preached it was a sacred duty to rob, murder and burn their fellow Christians who were preventing them from carrying out Pope Innocent's mandate to go to the Holy Land and redeem the Holy Sepulchre in the Holy City of Jerusalem. Religion is always ready to go to war. The Generals had nothing to do but to release the dogs and let them ravage the countryside. The folly was that they were destroying the fields and farms that would have fed them through the winter and deepening the rift between Greeks and Romans until it erupted like a volcano.

Where was Kit? Riding out of camp with the Sergeant and twenty men from St. Foy. He no longer feared being recognised, he was Kit his lordship's page and groom. He had volunteered to join the raiding party, Alaric had dared him and Robert approved and gave him a short sword. The boy should be blooded.

Their objectives were the villas of wealthy Jewish and Genoese merchants on the wooded slopes above the Bosporus. They were to pay for the muddle-headedness of Alexius and the Generals. The approach was civilised, over a well-bricked road through the trees. Kit had occasional glimpses of the narrow channel below, racing from where he did not know to where he did not know. Action is in the minute and in one place. He anticipated drawing his short sword and taking some valuables from an undeserving foreigner for a good cause. It was not going to be like the tower. If the tower was Kit's baptism in blood, this was to be his confirmation.

They did not hurry. The casual nature of the war suited the fact that there was no cause for it except folly. They deliberately allowed the inhabitants of the villas they were going to rob to escape. The first villa they came across was palatial, perhaps the country residence of a great merchant who lived in the city. It stood in a cultivated garden, two floors in the Byzantine style of opulent elegance, with a balcony looking over the Bosporus. It appeared to be deserted and the doors and windows were open. The men of St. Foy entered and destroyed everything they could not steal.

The Sergeant sent a party down to the cellars to take the winter stores of food and wine for the camp. They seized the things they recognised and scattered the rest, valuable oils and spices from China and Egypt were trodden underfoot. The others wandered casually through the salons taking their pick of the gold and silver objects on display. They tossed precious vases to each other and let them crash, tore down the silks and tapestries on the walls. They broke open chests and cupboards in search of jewels. They burnt books and manuscripts, maps and parchments, for their amusement. They killed a cat in case it was not a Christian.

Kit had gone upstairs. He did not want a treasure. He avoided the rich apartments and entered a room at the back of the villa, drawn to it by the simplicity of the doorway.

There was a table in the room and by it an old man with white hair and a white beard, wearing a white kaftan, was leaning over the body of a boy about Kit's age wrapped in the winding sheet of death. The old man turned to see who had intruded on his grief. He saw a figure with the red cross on its shoulder, cried out and as if to protect the boy started towards Kit with his hands stretched out. Kit drew the sword, more startled than afraid. The old man began to run towards him and he instinctively raised the sword to protect himself. He thought the old man would stop, but whether in the agony of grief or the fury of anger, he ran onto the sword which pierced his body with the sound of tearing cloth.

It had happened in a second. Kit was astounded. The old man fell back with the sword embedded in his body, wrenched out of Kit's hand. The flesh clung to it like a lover. There was no blood.

Kit stood for a moment that seemed to stretch from creation to the last judgement. Had he killed the old man or was he merely the instrument of a death desired? He was somewhere between Bishop and the Cross.

He left the dead with the dead. He heard the Sergeant shouting and went down, leaving the villa with the others.

When he returned to the camp Robert asked for the sword.

"My lord, I dropped it."

Robert laughed, "You boys!"

He was in a good mood. It was war.

Kit did not pray. He did not confess. He did not think about it. It had happened. It was war.

Much later it changed his life.

The memory of the old Jew sank into the cloaca of the brain where evil dreams are born.

As Dandolo had expected and perhaps hoped, the Greeks reacted violently to the depredation of the countryside, though he had not expected the violence to be directed at him. On a black night in December trumpets sounded the alarm in the crusader camp. The men turned out to meet an attack on land, but the watch were pointing towards the Venetian fleet in the Golden Horn. They lay in darkness but further up the Horn there was the glow of burning ships. At first Kit thought the Venetians must have captured some vessels and set them on fire but the Sergeant came up behind him.

"Fireships. It's an old trick. They fill a hulk with dry wood and rope soaked in tar and oil and set it on fire."

"Why?"

"It's not to warm their hands, son."

Kit saw why. The fireships were bearing down on the Venetians in the harbour. In the glimmer he could see the sailors like little black ants running up the rigging to set sail, jumping down into boats and barges, rowing out into the current to grapple with the fireships and tow them away from the fleet. He watched anxiously. Without the ships there was no way to reach the Holy Land. Others were thinking there was no way to go home. Venetian seamanship won the night. The fireships were towed safely past and released to drift into the Bosporus and out to sea. A few nights later there was a second attempt. This time the fireships were roped together to form a crescent of flames, but they proved to be nothing more dangerous than a spectacle.

The winter was not as cold as the winters in St. Foy. Kit slept in the stable with Thunderer a great black comforting presence, or in the pavilion where Lord Robert was the opposite. He ate where he could but less and less as the Generals' lack of foresight left the crusaders short of food. One day Thunderer's manger was empty. This was worse than his own plate. He went to the commissary for his sack of dry biscuit and then looked round the camp. There was a line of men outside a tent and he joined it and shuffled slowly forward with the others. After about an hour it was his turn and he pulled aside the curtain to see Poet sitting at a table counting a heap of sous.

"Kit! You didn't have to wait!"

Poet jumped up and seized hold of him.

"Kit my boy, you're looking a bit seedy. Look!" he turned to a fat man working amongst a pile of crates and barrels and Kit saw chicken coops. "It's Kit!"

Bishop came round and hugged him in turn. Then he held him at arm's length.

"He's put on a bit of weight."

"He's a growing lad," said Poet.

"Ah, Kit," said Bishop, "you should never have left us. We've found gold, except you can eat it."

"It's the dearest little fiddle in the world. Uncle Flyn never did it better."

"What are you doing, Poet?" Kit wanted to ask Bishop what he had been doing in the brothel but he thought he had better not.

It was Bishop who answered.

"Two sous an egg. Twenty a chicken. Thirty a bottle of wine."

If they had been his children he could not have been more proud.

"Tell us how much you want," said Poet.

"I'll have an egg please."

Bishop went and fetched him an egg. Kit waited hoping it was free but Poet said, "Two sous. I'll walk back with you."

Before he left the tent Kit looked back at Bishop. Bishop shook his head.

"God be with you Bishop." He thought God might do better than he could.

He walked with Poet. He carried the sack and Poet the egg.

"Where did you get it?" he asked.

"Where do you think? The Venetians sell it to us. They'd sell each other's mothers."

"I saw Bishop in the city."

"Kit, don't grow up. It's growing up causes all the trouble in the world."

"Have you thought of what happens if you don't?"

"I have, I have. You become a general."

They had reached the pavilion.

"Can I have my egg please?"

"Is that yours? I thought it was mine."

Thunderer ate his biscuits, Kit ate his egg.

He could not stop wondering where the egg came from. Poet had said the Venetians, but where could they have found an egg? Then he remembered how Bishop had shaken his head. That is where the egg came from with the wine and the chickens and what else. The kitchen of the brothel! But why had he lied to Poet? To conceal that he was playing on both sides, he had said he was neutral. Lying was natural to them all, but so was cheating and stealing and Poet had no objection to either. Why was Poet different? He was Irish. Where was Ireland? Kit had no idea. But, he thought, it must be a place of great commitment because Poet was the only one who was keeping the oath they took in St. Foy. Ireland must be full of saints and dreamers.

So far the Greeks had shown they had little inclination for a fight. The attacks by fireships had not involved any danger for the perpetrators unless they burnt themselves. The crusader raids on the countryside had no effect on the city except to infuriate the citizens.

"They're ready to burst," said Deuce, "but they've got no one to prick them. They say Alexius is doing nothing because we're the only friends he's got."

Deuce was in high favour, being in and out of Montferrat's pavilion when he was not being in and out of Constantinople on his donkey.

"He's safe," said Deuce, "as long as the Varangian Guard stick to him."

"Who?" asked Kit.

"Your friend Alexius. He's as safe as a man in a cage of lions, until the first one bites him."

On a dark morning later in December the trumpets sounded the alarm and the crusaders assembled in their divisions. Kit armed Thunderer and ran him to Lord Robert's pavilion. The Sergeant had paraded the company and all around men were tripping over tent ropes, archers were stringing their bows, lords were calling for their squires and pages to help them into their armour.

The word passed round. The watch had heard the sounds of many horses, the chink of bridles, the clang of metal. There was movement from the city gate nearest the Blachernae palace on the far side of the Golden Horn. A force of crusaders had been stationed there to protect the Venetian shipping from an attack by land. There was a part of Count Hugh's division and about a hundred lords and knights with their squires and pages. Kit knew that Alaric was amongst them.

There was no time for the army to march to the bridge to reach them before the enemy.

It grew lighter and the crusaders lining the banks of the Golden Horn could see the coming battle under the walls of the city.

"There is the blue banner of Count Hugh of St. Pol," said the Sergeant.

There is Alaric, thought Kit.

There must have been a thousand Greeks and mercenaries and four troops of cavalry. They were led by a man Lord Robert claimed later he recognised by his thickset eyebrows, but he could not pronounce his name. It was Mourtzouphlus.

They saw the lords lower their lances and the foot soldiers move forward. They heard the cry from across the water: "Charge!"

They held their breath and stared as the thin ranks of crusaders moved at a gathering pace towards the mass of men and horses. Kit wished he was among them and felt the thudding of the hooves and the thumping of his heart, heard the snort of horses and clash of armour and saw the wall of the enemy begin to crumble and crack with the impact of lance, shield, man and horse and be swept aside, or trampled, or fall to be despatched by the soldiers running after.

So it was. The Greeks turned and galloped back towards the gate. Once there, they were in range of their own bowmen and archers on the wall. Mourtzouphlus had stood until the last before he joined the flood. His horse faltered, he fell and would have been killed or taken but for the arrows and bolts pouring down from the wall.

Alaric had done well. He had followed his lord and when his lance was broken handed him his sword. He had fought hand-to-hand with his short sword and dagger. He had been cut on the shoulder near the cross.

"Stop fussing," he told Kit, "you're worse than a woman." He did not know how bad a woman could be and was merely repeating something he had heard. Kit did not know that and wondered if womanising and heroism went together as it did in Aimery.

Alexius was not a hero but then he did not like women.

Alexius was not a hero in his own capital city. He was confined to the Blachernae palace and protected by the Varangian Guard. The grand families who were usually involved in the affairs of state retreated to their mansions or left the city for their estates, blaming Alexius for the loss of empire and fearing for Constantinople. Power drifted down like powder into the streets.

"They're the out-of-work, the don't-want-to-work, the there-might-be-something-in-it-for-me's and some who really care," said Deuce. "The usual lot. The good people have shut up their shops, locked their doors and are waiting to see."

"To see what?" asked Kit.

"That's it," said Deuce, "what?"

He had reported the effect of the rout of the Greeks to Montferrat and the Generals. The simmering discontent had boiled over into sporadic rioting and defacing of Roman inscriptions and monuments, anything that reminded them of the crusaders' presence over the Golden Horn.

"They'd make old Eyebrows emperor but he's too crafty to show his hand." Nobody could pronounce Mourtzouphlus.

"It's cold out here," said Kit.

"It's getting hot in there." Deuce nodded at the grey city under the grey January sky.

There was nothing the crusaders could do but wait and hope Alexius would last long enough to keep his promises and pay his debts. Then they could sail to the Holy Land in March and be in Jerusalem in August and home in December.

To the Generals, all the twisting and turning of the pilgrimage appeared to have been the unavoidable progression of events they could not possibly have foreseen. Their heads were caves of dragons, a dragon of Christian virtue, a dragon of martial bravery, a dragon of ignorance of anything outside their castles, a dragon of hope, a dragon of despair, a dragon of greed and ambition. Each one jousted for the prize, none won for long, all served to destroy the men under their care and command.

Alaric wanted to go back again into the city. He was determined to finish what he had barely begun, the more so since the fight. He was worried he might be killed before it ever happened.

"I shan't go with you," said Kit.

"Good."

"It's dangerous."

"You're not going."

"Yes I am."

A boatman rowed them across the Golden Horn at dusk. They had smeared their white faces to look like chimney sweeps. The gate was open and unguarded. The streets were deserted. Alaric led the way to the business quarter and Kit followed, wondering what it could be that attracted him so strongly. Whatever it was it flopped. The street was empty, the house closed up, the windows shuttered. Alaric used a word Kit had never heard before, even in the company of Bishop and the others. Doubtless Alaric had heard it from one of his noble acquaintances. Then he said he was going to find out where everybody was. Kit protested.

"Let's go back!"

"An Alaric de Clairon never retreats."

Kit had to run after him. They caught up with some stragglers from the crowd that was moving slowly through the streets and squares in the centre of the city towards the great cathedral shining like a silver scimitar spanning the sky. They were carried along by a throng of Greeks, Armenians, Bulgars, Romans, the citizens of a Byzantine empire beginning to disintegrate even now, cracked by the crusade. There were already three emperors, one in exile, one insane, one in confinement and this ungovernable mob was about to create another. Kit and Alaric were being swept along by history. In St. Sophia they were jammed in amongst a sweating press of humanity stinking of sour wine and garlic. The walls glistened with grease and Christ hanging from the dome looked down on His people through a cloud of foul breath. The cynosure of all eyes was the golden-pillared tribune raised before the glittering altar. The old white-bearded Patriarch, his tiara crooked on his head and his dalmatic torn in the haste of dressing, was pushed up and stood visibly shaking between two senators. On the other side of the tribune, a young man apparently taken from his bed was waiting, glancing nervously from a burly escort to the mass below. A gold tiara was produced from somewhere, the young man knelt and the Patriarch placed it on his head. The crowd was shouting and in the racket, Kit heard the name "Canabus." The new emperor was Canabus. Alaric was tugging his sleeve.

"We've got to get back!"

Retreat was now essential and not easy. There was a solid scrum of flesh between them and the street. Kit pushed Alaric and whispered, "Fight me." He began swinging his arms and shouting, "Come on! Come on!" Alaric had to defend himself. The people nearest them pushed back to escape the blows and made a circle. Alaric angrily thrust Kit to the ground and fell on top of him. Protests arose, "Fighting in church!" "Throw them out!" "Young ruffians!" Some men pulled them apart, the crowd gave way and they were marched out and told to get off! They ran back to the boat.

Kit had not been in the company of rogues for nothing.

They were stopped at the perimeter of the camp by the watch. Two black-faced boys were suspect. They were brought before the Sergeant-at-Arms.

"What's your name?"

"Alaric de Clairon, page to Count Hugh of St. Pol."

"And you?"

"Kit, sir. Page to Lord Robert of St. Foy."

"I've never heard of him. What's your other name?"

Kit was silent.

"You heard me. What's your father's name?"

Kit could not speak and Alaric saved him.

"His name is Chretien ... de Quatre, the king's marshal."

"Why didn't he say so?"

"He didn't wish to humble you, Sergeant."

They ran to Count Hugh's pavilion. Alaric told his story, the mob had proclaimed a new emperor and there was no word of Alexius.

Montferrat and the Generals were woken. A message was sent to the Doge.

A council was called for the morning. Kit was leaving when Alaric stopped him.

"It's no disgrace to be a bastard. It's obvious your father was a gentleman, otherwise you wouldn't be in my company. Good night."

Kit returned to the stable. Thunderer turned his great head and eyed him reproachfully. Kit had woken him up.

"Excuse me, my Lord Cheval," said Kit, "allow me to introduce myself, I am Chretien de Quatre, bastard." He giggled.

The council met in Montferrat's pavilion and almost at once were told a deputy had arrived from the Blachernae palace with a message from the Emperor Alexius. They stood and waited and stared as the deputy entered - it was Mourtzouphlus!

Naïve to the last, Alexius had sent the one man in Constantinople he could trust the least. Perhaps he thought he could compromise him by sending him to the crusader camp, perhaps in his vanity he thought he was above fate, perhaps he did not think at all. Mourtzouphlus bowed deeply, congratulated the Generals on their success in slaughtering so many of his compatriots and begged their acceptance of a plea from his master the Emperor Alexius.

They let him stand while they sat down.

Alexius re-affirmed all the promises he had made and assured them, with the usual Byzantine elaboration, that he would provide the money and resources to allow them to sail to the Holy Land in March. Mourtzouphlus turned to Montferrat, who had involved Alexius in the crusade from the beginning. In return, would his excellency send a small force of crusaders into the city to remove the imposter Canabus from St. Sophia and dispel his mob of supporters?

"They could hardly believe it," said Deuce, sitting on the banks of the Golden Horn with Kit and Poet the next day. "They were like kids going to the fair. They were being given Constantinople on a platter."

The Generals had agreed with alacrity and alacrity had never meant so much. Mourtzouphlus took his leave with a smile, he had been given the key to the empire.

"I went back with him in his suite," said Deuce.

"Better than in his privy," added Poet.

"He went straight to the barracks of the Varangian Guard and told them Alexius was planning to betray them and hand the city over to the crusaders. He said Alexius had broken his oath as Emperor to defend the city and that released them from theirs to defend him. For which they would be rewarded of course."

"What happened?"

"You don't want to know."

"I do."

"They marched to St. Sophia and drove away the mob. Canabus held on to the altar for a bit until they dragged him out and cut his head off."

Kit closed his eyes and saw the reluctant young man being crowned and now uncrowned.

"They went into the great palace and found old Isaac."

"Ah, the poor old gentleman," said Poet, "at least he didn't see what was coming."

Not Alexius, thought Kit, please not Alexius!

"Last night," said Deuce. Kit was looking at him pitifully. "I'm sorry, Kit."

"Don't drop your tears on him. Without him we'd have been in Jerusalem by now." Poet was not of the sentimental school.

"How?" Kit hoped it had been brave and noble.

"Strangled," said Deuce.

"Ah," said Poet, "it would have spoiled his complexion."

Having murdered three emperors in twenty-four hours Mourtzouphlus was Emperor.

Kit wept.

The Generals had been outplayed at their own game. They were worse off than before because there was no guarantee Mourtzouphlus would keep to the treaty signed by Alexius. The city was showing more signs of resistance, many of the gates were bricked up and the walls broken down by the Venetians were rebuilt. The fields and farms within foraging distance had been stripped of provisions and the crusaders were going hungry. Bishop's little tent of luxuries was empty.

"He never got them from the Venetians," protested Poet.

Kit thought, he won't get them from the brothel either.

He saw Bishop.

To provide the army with food, the Generals made a plan to send a force of mounted crusaders to raid a prosperous town on the Black Sea about two days' ride away. A section of Count Baldwin's division from Flanders was ordered to attack the town of Phileas and come away with as many cattle and as much grain and fodder, food and clothing, as they could. Thirty lords and squires and a hundred sergeants rode out of the camp on a morning in February. Kit was watching and was surprised to see Bishop wearing a helmet, chain-mail hauberk and carrying a banner with the yellow cross of Flanders, riding a squat wagon-horse. He felt sorry for the citizens of Phileas.

There was no word of the expedition for three days and then the rumour spread that the new emperor had led an army from the city to intercept the Flanders forces on the way back. The boatmen and fishermen who crossed the Golden Horn brought stories of four thousand picked soldiers, carrying the sacred icon of the Virgin that had protected Constantinople for a thousand years, waiting to intercept the crusaders. A relief force was sent out. Another day went by and there was still no word.

Kit was up early with Thunderer when he saw a herd of cows coming over the hill driven by four or five weary men with yellow crosses on their shoulders. Was that all that was left of Flanders? He rode up to them. One was a young farm boy who had taken the oath in a Flemish hamlet with his heart full of God. He looked up at Kit with an old face.

"Victory," he said.

It was. Bishop told them about it later. He had ridden back on a glossy palfrey with his pockets full of trinkets. His helmet was dented and his dagger blunted. He shared a stolen flask of Black Sea wine with Kit and Poet in a tent he had commandeered.

"A hundred and thirty," he kept saying, "a hundred and thirty against thousands and they had the advantage of surprise. We were burdened by the stuff we'd taken and they came upon us in a wood. Well, we had eight bowmen and we put them in front but they had no time to shoot. The lords threw down their lances and we grappled hand-to-hand."

"Where were you?" asked Kit.

"Why lad, in the middle. The lords were wheeling round as they do in the tourneys, hacking with their long swords, whilst the squires were watching their backs and pricking the footmen with their daggers."

"What were you doing, Bishop?"

"In a minute. The sergeants were doing deeds worthy of Achilles, pike to pike, swing, hold, thrust!"

"For sure he was writing it all down," said Poet.

Bishop looked lordly.

"It was a fair fight and we were going to lose, so I slipped off my little horse, I drew my misericord and dodged beneath the Greek horses' bellies, slitting their hamstrings."

He took out the long thin dagger and caressed it. Kit was nearly sick. Bishop had not finished.

"And when their riders had fallen and lay like beetles on their backs ... whip!"

He cut an imaginery throat.

"If he'd only tell us the truth, Kit," said Poet, "he'd admit he won the battle himself entirely."

"What happened then?"

"They ran Kit, they ran and we charged after them and many were struck down. Eyebrows himself was there."

"The Emperor?"

"In his golden helmet and more, he was holding the icon in his bosom and he flung it down on the ground to stop us."

Kit gasped.

"Did it?"

"It did."

"The sacred icon of the Virgin?"

"The sacred jewels round the sacred icon of the Virgin."

"You didn't!"

"Unfortunately I was on foot."

There were cattle and clothing, the crusaders only had the clothes they came in, stores and provisions for a month. It was February and they were sailing in March.

It was a victory but it did not win the city. Mourtzouphlus was still alive and claiming he had won and that the icon was safely in his vaults. He had shown valour and determination. The citizens of Constantinople were more concerned with peace in their city than with war outside it. Behind their massive walls they bore the hardships and dangers of their soldiers stoically. The war was an inconvenience rather than a concern, like a distant roll of thunder, until the fury of the storm burst on them.

The Generals were more concerned. The Doge had sent them a message. Mourtzouphlus had asked for a truce so that they could meet and discuss terms for peace. He had agreed. Montferrat and the Generals knew the lease of the Venetian fleet was up and the ships could sail at any moment. They did not trust Dandolo.

This was an element of the crusade and perhaps of all crusades. Each party has two purposes, God's and its own, the ideal and the sordid reality. Therefore one does not trust the other. Every crusade in history has ended in division and disaster. God's cause is incomprehensible, man's insufferable.

The Generals expected Dandolo was about to betray them, take money from the Emperor and leave them stranded in Constantinople. The meeting was to take place the next day at a monastery on the banks of the Golden Horn. The Doge would be in his galley and the Emperor on the jetty. They contrived a hasty plan to disrupt the meeting and capture Mourtzouphlus. It did not worry them that their ally had agreed to a flag of truce. They regarded Mourtzouphlus as a renegade traitor who had murdered his lord and broken the feudal code by which they lived. He was a fox who could be hunted and killed.

Lord Robert was given the whip. He chose a small body of mounted men and rode out before dawn to wait in ambush behind the monastery. They were lightly armed and relied upon surprise and speed to scatter the Emperor's bodyguard. Kit was on foot with his hand over Thunderer's nostrils to stop him snorting, which he did when he was excited. He could see a stretch of water and the jetty.

He whispered to Robert, "They're coming."

The Doge's galley slid into view, the rowers shipping their oars so it could moor at the jetty.

"He's here."

Mourtzouphlus appeared from the monastery with a dozen Varangians. Kit could not hear what they were saying and it did not matter as Robert twitched the reins, Thunderer's head went up, Kit's hand slipped and they were off! Kit saw the Emperor disappearing, the Varangians running and the Doge raise his hands in despair at the folly of his friends.

There was no way Robert could storm the monastery and the farce ended with a monk coming out and asking them to go away.

"It's everyone's fault but ours," said Alaric.

It was a God-given day in February and it was not raining. They were riding out together. Alaric had wanted to go to the grove but Kit had forbidden it, Alaric did not need any more excitement. There was a hiatus in the crusade that looked as if it might develop into complete decomposition.

"I was with Lord Hugh in council. It's hopeless, Chretien."

"Who?"

"You, you idiot. I can't call you Kit, it's common. He said since Alexius was dead there was no hope Eyebrows would keep to the treaty and that means no money, no ships, no food, no Holy Land. I blame Alexius!"

Kit saw Alexius, tragic and beautiful.

"I blame that old blind fool Dandolo."

Kit saw the Doge, wise and brave, sitting in his chair under the walls of the city.

"I blame the dumb idiots who took the oath without the means to keep it."

Kit saw the dead at the foot of the ladder.

"I blame …"

Kit shouted, "Why don't you blame yourself, Alaric? Why don't you blame Lord Hugh and the Generals who could have taken us to Jerusalem if they'd wanted to, but they took Alexius's money instead!"

Alaric snatched Mercury's head back nearly breaking his jaw.

"Weren't you taught your lord can do no wrong? And his lord can do no wrong? And the king can do no wrong? Because they were put over us by God who can do no wrong!"

Kit looked sheepish.

"Haven't you any loyalty? Any chivalry? Any honour? No! You haven't because you're some peasant's bastard … Kit!"

Alaric spurred Mercury on and rode as far apart from Kit as he could until they reached the camp. Then he turned to Kit.

"You're no company for a gentleman!"

He jerked the reins. Mercury had had enough and kicked up his heels spraying Alaric with an unspeakable porridge of mud and excrement. Alaric rode proudly away as if it suited him.

Conditions in the camp had deteriorated quickly and every crusader and the tent he lived in was covered in a film of slime. Groundsheets split and leaked, canvas let in the rain, cooking pots slipped from wet hands, the fires beneath them smoked and spat and seemed to take more heat out of the air than they put into it. The provisions taken from Phileas were exhausted and it was rumoured some of the wagon-horses had mysteriously disappeared. There was the sour-sweet smell of boiling horse-hock everywhere. Kit went to see Thunderer was safe.

"Don't blame circumstances Kit, profit from them."

Bishop was in a philosophical mood. The tent was warm and dry, his plate was full and his glass was empty. He filled it.

"Look at them from the other side."

"We should have been in Jerusalem by now."

"That's a hot and dangerous place Kit," said Poet, "didn't they murder Christ Himself in Jerusalem?"

"That's why we're going."

Deuce leant forward.

"I heard the other day they knew all the time we were coming here."

The others turned to him.

"Montferrat knew about Alexius before we started. Alexius had been to see the Pope and the Pope said no so he went to see Montferrat."

"You can't blame the Pope," said Kit.

"The deal was to go to Jerusalem all right, but to stop off at Constantinople on the way and make Alexius emperor. Why else was there a clause in the treaty that he'd make the Greek Church submit to the Pope unless they knew he was going to fix it?"

"So his Holy Innocence said no when he meant yes," said Poet, "that's beautiful."

Deuce had more to say.

"It wasn't the only time. Remember the two letters at Zara? The excommunication that never was? The Pope wanted Jerusalem but he wanted Constantinople first."

Kit was not convinced.

"The Generals made all the decisions."

Bishop was portentous.

"Kit my boy, battles are won by heroes, not generals. Look what I did at Phileas."

"They fight like us."

"They do Kit, they're brave enough. It behoves them as they say. But they don't have a brain between them."

At that moment the Generals might have agreed with Bishop because they had just decided to go and see Enrico Dandolo, Doge of Venice, to ask him what to do.

Kit thought the Doge looked happy. He was standing behind Lord Robert's chair, wearing his tabard embroidered with Robert's armorial bearings, in case someone was not sure of his breeding and connections. Kit was looking straight at the Doge in his vermilion chair in his state-room in the vermilion galley. The Generals were seated in a circle. Alaric stood behind Lord Hugh refusing to look at Kit. Dandolo waited for someone to speak and when nobody did he spoke himself.

"You are in a hole, my lords."

They all spoke together.

"You got us into it by asking too much money for the ships."

"You kept us sitting on a sandbank in Venice."

"You kept demanding to be paid like a gondolier."

"You made us go to Zara to rob it for you."

"You made sure we dealt with Alexius and you had half of it."

"You brought us here for your own purposes."

"You were planning something with Mour … Moo …"

Robert gave up.

Dandolo waited for the clamour to subside.

"Would you like a little cold collation? No? I wanted to see the Emperor Mourtzouphlus to persuade him to keep the treaty you made with the unfortunate Alexius. He will not now."

Montferrat leant forward.

"What do you want us to do?"

This was the moment Dandolo had been waiting for since he first heard about the crusade.

"My friends, I want you to occupy Constantinople and annex the entire Byzantine empire."

They were shocked into silence. It was far beyond anything they had thought of before. They had made Alexius emperor in order to reach the Holy Land, they would defeat Mourtzouphlus and put up a puppet emperor for the same end, but here was the opportunity to take the empire for themselves!

Kit did not understand what was happening. Dandolo had said something that stunned the Generals. Occupy Constantinople, not besiege it take what you want and go away, but occupy! That meant to stay. To abandon the crusade. Never to go to the Holy Land. To become kings and rulers of an empire. They must say no! Their oaths, their chivalry, their honour, their loyalty to Christ must make them say no.

Montferrat spoke first.

"The whole empire?"

"After you've taken Constantinople."

"All of us?" Robert spoke loudly, as if suddenly aware he might be a king.

"Of course," said Dandolo, "except me. I will return to Venice," he paused, "with half the city for my people. We do not want a province or a kingdom."

Kit thought, he is the wisest man in the room. He knows these lords. He knows they think in terms of land, of lineage, of titles, of families. They wore them on their banners and their shields. They would all want to be kings.

Dandolo continued, "And for Christ whom we all worship you will bring the holiness of Papal rule to these barbarians. You will fulfil your obligations to the Pope who will release you from your oaths. You will redeem the sacred relics hoarded in the churches and abbeys for centuries and give them to the world. The pieces of the Cross, the bones of the apostles, the veil of the Virgin, the cloak of Christ stained with His blood. Then you will go to the Holy Land if you wish. All this will be at your disposal. As emperor your powers will be infinite."

Montferrat asked casually, "Who will be emperor?"

"You must decide amongst yourselves. Not me, I assure you."

They glanced at each other, weighing up their chances.

Baldwin spoke up, "We don't need to decide now."

They rose and crowded round the old man to kiss his hands as if the empire was already in theirs. Behind Robert's chair Kit was witnessing a crime of universal proportions being plotted by decent men in the name of God. They were prepared to repudiate their oaths to go in arms to the Holy Sepulchre and to betray Christ for an empire. It was too big for him to grasp. Jerusalem dwindled to the Jerusalem in the corner of the rood screen in St. Foy. St. Foy was a garden plot. France would fit into one of the provinces of the empire. The words of Dandolo, few enough, had expanded into a history of the world glorifying the lives of these empty men. Kit reeled and fainted.

Robert thought when I'm king I'll get another page.

The Generals' elation evaporated as they returned to the camp and saw their dirty and disheartened men doing as little as possible. They had primed them with promises and now had to persuade them to forget them, renege on their oaths and forgo two years' absence, hardship and suffering. For what? If they had looked behind them they could have seen the walls of the city filling the sky. How could they convince them, or threaten them, or offer them? They turned to the priests whose business it was to convince, threaten and offer.

For the next few days, black-garbed ministers were seen scuttling between the tents like beetles on a dung-heap. Kit received a sermon. He was grooming Thunderer and compared his glossy hide to the priest's drab stuff. He learnt it was his duty to oust the murderous Mourtzouphlus, priests were used to long names and to punish his supporters who prayed a false doctrine in a foreign tongue. In truth an assault on Constantinople was a crusade in itself and all the benefits of dying in a siege of Jerusalem would apply to a siege of Constantinople. In truth the Greeks were worse than Saracens because they pretended to be Christians and if Christ ever came to Constantinople He would surely be crucified all over again. Kit did not faint but Thunderer was glossier than he had ever been. In the camp those who believed believed, those who did not believe had nowhere else to go and nothing else to do and Bishop was in heaven.

It was March, the month the crusaders should have been at sea on the way to the Holy Land and instead they were preparing to besiege a city they had failed to take six months earlier. The sun was shining but the star that had led them from the towns and fields of France had gone out. In spite of the priests' assurances Christ was not here. They would fight because their lords were going to fight. How many campaigns and wars have been fought on that fatal premiss?

Louis of St. Blois contracted some other germ from the meeting on the galley and went down with a fever. Lord Robert was put in temporary command of the division and spent hours in conference with the Generals.

"They're planning the campaign," said Kit.

Deuce grinned contemptuously.

"What then?"

"They're splitting up the empire between them"

"They would, they would," said Poet, "we spill the blood and they split up the corpse."

Bishop thought there would be a toe or two for them. Deuce disagreed.

"Every man will have to swear on the Bible to give up any gold or silver or even a piece of cloth worth more than five sous, to the Provost and he mustn't touch a woman or her garment or a monk or he'll be hanged."

"What would I do with a monk?" asked Bishop.

Kit knew.

"You're a wonderful man, Deuce," said Poet, "have you got the cloak of invisibility?"

"Montferrat's squire has a mistress. I think they share her, they're Italian. She's Greek, she's a spy, she talks to me. They're going to choose an emperor and a new patriarch, the Venetians are going to own half the city and the others are going to have to fight for what little kingdoms and provinces they can get."

"What about the crusade? What about the Holy Sepulchre in Jerusalem?"

They looked at Kit and shook their heads. Deuce was the kindest.

"Grow up Kit. It's a pity but grow up."

Kit had grown up more than they knew.

In the month that followed, what compassion the crusaders might have had was burned up in a growing hatred of the walls they saw every day but which now seemed to have surrounded them and stopped them from their purpose which had been to crusade and not to destroy a Christian city. The end to which they were now destined itself destroyed the faith in which they had started.

Kit felt a guilt that raised the ghost of the old Jew he had killed. Crime could be unintended or the end of good intentions. All around the camp the men were preparing to renew the war against Constantinople.

Robert was constantly sending messages which the sergeants were ignoring and getting on with their business. Local houses were broken up for timbers to build siege engines and stones to hurl from them. The sappers built "cats" or "sows" as they called them, wooden pigsties on wheels, under which they would pick at the huge stones of the walls until they were crushed by smaller ones from above. Men built more ladders to make more grave markers.

Kit's eyes had lost the stars that had once shone in them. He saw the fatuity of the Generals who were determined to make the same mistakes twice.

One evening after a day when both Robert and Thunderer had been particularly irksome, he was sitting with Bishop and Poet watching the setting sun turn the Golden Horn to gold.

Poet pointed to the Venetian ships in the harbour.

"Those Venicers are clever fellows, they're topping up their flying bridges to reach above the towers."

"I wouldn't go up in one of those for a thousand silver marks," said Bishop.

"What would you do?" asked Kit. Bishop did not seem to belong to any part of the army.

"The gates," said Bishop. "They bricked up the gates. With bricks."

"You're a poet Bishop," said Poet, "you see things other men don't."

Alaric avoided him. They were often in the same pavilion where the Generals were meeting, but nobility can be blind when it wants to be. Kit could not stop looking at Alaric, but Kit did not know his place. He had never had a place, only a bucket.

He spent as much time as he could with Thunderer.

His body disturbed him. Sometimes he felt it did not belong to him. It had a subversive life of its own. He had only lived amongst men. The old cleaner might have been a man for all it mattered. The presence of men, the talk of men, the smell of men, the habits of men, had made him no longer a boy but a man. His body did not agree, which disturbed him. He did not want it.

Ten days before Palm Sunday was Friday 9th April 1204.

Kit woke before dawn. He felt unwell, ill at ease, heartsick. Thunderer had been restless all night. He resisted Kit's attempts to put on his coat of mail, he chewed his reins, he stamped his great hooves deliberately near Kit's toes. Kit's own dressing-up was tiresome, the tunic refused to button, the tabard was heavy and hot, he hated the cap with the feather. As he hung the dagger from his belt he hoped he would not have to use it.

Outside, the grey dawn touched the ghostlike figures emerging from the tents. Kit looked to where the Venetian ships were moored in a long line waiting to carry the army across the Golden Horn. Behind them the black outline of the city lay like the jagged back of some huge ancient monster. Candles were burning in the pavilion where the Squire was struggling to get Lord Robert into his armour. As General of a division Robert was overloaded with responsibilities without the staffs that supported the great lords. The men had to be got ready for embarkation, the siege engines and ladders to be loaded on the ships, the disposition of the division to be determined once it had been landed on the shore between the sea and the walls.

Kit went outside and sat next to the Sergeant.

"Officers," said the Sergeant, "are never wrong. They're not often right but they're never wrong."

"We ran away last time," said Kit.

"By the same mark son, we may retreat but we never run away."

"We're alone this time."

The Sergeant contemplated Kit for a long moment.

"I'll give you a good tip lad. If you have to fight fight like the devil. If you don't mean it, you'll get it."

Drums were beating and the crusaders formed up in their divisions. A priest stood in front of each division to take the sacrament on behalf of the men. It was enough to witness it as to partake of it. Kit saw with surprise that the priest was Aimery, wearing a surplice over his armour. It was rumoured Aimery had been in the hospital at Scutari recovering from a local disease. As Aimery raised the cup the men's heads were down and they fidgeted and shuffled as if they were embarrassed or ashamed. It suddenly struck Kit that the actions and words were meaningless, almost sacrilegious. Christ was not in the sacrament! Christ was not there! Christ was in Jerusalem!

There was no joy in the marching down to the ships, the banners were limp, some of the men had covered up their crosses. If they were not going to fight for Christ they were not going to fight like the devil.

It took six hours or more to move the army, reduced in numbers as it was, across the Golden Horn. When they were there they looked insignificant in the shadow of the walls. The galleys and transports sailed down almost half a mile away to where they could abut on the walls within reach of the flying bridges.

Then they waited. What heart they had dried up. On the wall over their heads flew a flag with the watchword of the city, "Jesus Christ the Victor". Constantinople was stronger than before. Mourtzouphlus had shown spirit. They had heightened the towers and built up stocks of projectiles for the mangonels to hurl with their swinging arms at the ships and men below. There was steam rising which the attackers did not understand until they were showered with Greek fire, a fierce mixture of burning oil, tar and sand. Whilst the citizens might wait until they could see which side won, the mercenaries and Varangian Guards had personal reasons to defend the city. They would fight as long as the walls were not breached.

Robert set up his standard on a rise opposite the Blachernae palace from where he could see along the wall to where it abutted on the sea about half a mile away. The sails of the Venetians were just visible. He waited for the trumpet to sound the charge. His men would advance under a curtain of arrows to set the ladders against the wall and endure a burst of rocks and burning oil. The sappers would roll the "cats" to the base of the wall and wield picks against stone twenty feet deep.

Kit stood behind Robert with his shield and sword. The men of Blois, like those of St. Foy, were feudal serfs, farmhands, labourers, who had seen their companions slaughtered in the first assault. What gave them courage now that they were no longer fighting for Christ but for profit? He answered himself, fear. It was the opposite to faith. Fear is a great instigator. One fear cancels out another. Fear can have a terrible attraction. Men are the only creatures who go willingly into danger. Death is another country.

It was midday. The sun was high. Kit heard the trumpet. He feared to fight. He feared to run away. He knew what he would see, he saw it, he was sick.

There was a painting in the chapel at St. Foy, very old and grimy, half rubbed out. It showed three crosses on a hill. The old lord had brought it back from the Holy Land. Kit had asked one of the nuns who they were.

"The one in the middle is Jesus, Kitty."

"Who are the others?"

"The floor's still dirty!"

The good nun did not like thieves. Kit knew some thieves. One he loved.

He heard the sounds of cheers and jeers coming from the wall. Greek soldiers were standing on the parapets and towers, waving their weapons. Some of them turned their backs on the crusaders running away and dropped their breeches baring their buttocks.

The charge, like a wave crashing against a cliff, had fallen back leaving human detritus on the beach. It had taken barely an hour.

Robert was shouting for him.

"Message for the Doge!"

As he rode through the shattered ranks the men hardly looked up at him. There were defenders on the walls all the way down to where the land narrowed to within arrow-shot and he had to dismount and leave Thunderer with a nervous Venetian sailor. Skiffs were plying to and from the galleys and transports which had been becalmed and unable to grapple with the walls. Their sails drooped, some ripped by the rocks from the mangonels in the towers.

Kit waited to be rowed to the Doge's galley and saw the nearest ship, a giant transport with a flying bridge, caught in a wayward breeze that was taking it back to the wall. The sailors were climbing in the shrouds working frantically to lower the sail. In shallow water the ship began to roll, tilting the bridge nearer and nearer to a tower where the defenders were armed and ready. The sail was lowered and Kit could see the mast and the bridge clear against the blue sky. The end of the bridge was no more than ten feet away from the top of the tower.

There was someone on the bridge. Kit's heart leapt. He had seen him there before, with a rope around his neck. Poet had said then that he would be the first man to cross the bridge and fight for Christ. He had no sword or weapon and looked small and vulnerable. What did he mean to do?

The ship rolled back and the gap between bridge and tower widened. Kit closed his eyes and prayed, but when he opened them again the mast was swinging across the sky and the gap was closing. Poet moved unsteadily, nearly losing his balance, until he came to the end of the bridge just as it nearly touched the tower.

Kit prayed God move but Poet jumped. He fell against the side of the tower, the Greeks reached out to save him, he fell again and dropped and touched the wall and spun and died on the rocks below.

Why?

What had become so unbearable in the world that Poet wanted to leave it? Love? Grief? Death?

Poor Gentleman had died of love.

The old Jew had died of grief.

Did Poet die because death had become unbearable?

What was a crusade? Poet had said it was "to tell a foreign party what to do and kill him if he doesn't do it and then we go back home."

Murder for a cause and walk away.

Is that what God wanted? What Christ wanted?

Kit felt a surge of fierce resentment against God. Against Christ.

A little love does not go far, a little hate goes a long long way.

"The true Lord and Governor of the world has chastised the Romans with the scourge of his mercy so that all those who are sensible enough to face the facts, instead of engaging in obstinate debate may not abandon the true religion under pressure of the circumstances of the moment, but may adhere to it more loyally in confidence of eternal life."

"What did it mean?" asked Kit.

"What God usually means," said Bishop, "Don't argue with me or I'll do it again."

Bishop had decided to rejoin Lord Robert's company and they had just been given a sermon. The camp was a bee-hive of obstinate debate and the

Generals had ordered the priests to smoke it out. They quoted St. Augustine which usually worked to obfuscate matters.

The circumstances would not go away. The Generals were continually in council and Kit had time to think. He had left St. Foy bravely. He had fallen among thieves and found that they were just like other men. He had loved and lost and loved and lost again. He had been carried along by circumstances until he came to Constantinople. He had kept faith with Christ and that faith had been fatally compromised by circumstances. He could not forgive circumstances. Could he forgive Christ? Yes, if Christ wanted Constantinople instead of Jerusalem he would give Christ Constantinople or die. It was this perversity that achieved what St. Augustine could not achieve, although the saint would have smiled because he believed the end justified the means. But in Christ the means was the end. Kit had been here before but this time he was angry. It was an anger born of frustration and broken promises that men felt throughout the camp. They were angry with God, they would show God, then God would forgive them.

The Generals decided that, in the circumstances, the only course of action was the one that had failed twice before. God had brought them to this stage. They ordered the priests to exhort the men to greater efforts and to encourage them they banished all the women in the camp. There were some loose women but a lot of them were tied to their jobs as washerwomen and cooks and even more to the men who had picked them up on the march and who were honest wives. They were put aboard a ship and taken away, many never to see their husbands again. The anger this aroused provoked a furious activity as if there was a new crusade - to punish Constantinople instead of God - to fight like the devil.

As an incentive to fight, revenge is as good as religion. There were two days of furious industry to prepare for the next storm. The peals of the armourers' anvils rang round the camp accompanied by the hammers of the sappers nailing wet cowhides onto their "cats" and "sows" to ward off Greek fire. More stones were collected and more wood piled up for ladders. Men moved purposefully and the Sergeants wondered what had happened to them.

Kit found Lord Robert in a good mood.

"I shan't want Thunderer, I'm going to fight on foot."

"You can't leave him, my lord, he'll kick down the stable."

"Well bring him but keep him out of danger."

"I must be with you Lord Robert."

Robert looked at him with interest for the first time.

"Let the farrier look after him, he's used to being kicked."

"Yes my lord."

"Kit, is that your name Kit? Take my second hauberk."

"For you my lord?"

"No my boy, for you. It will fit you, you've filled out."

Kit was in the stable trying on the hauberk when he was hissed.

"Did you steal it?" asked Deuce.

"Lord Robert gave it me."

"You'll be a gentleman next Kit. You won't talk to me."

"I will Deuce."

"A spy's a despicable thing, nobody trusts a spy. A spy's worse than a thief, he doesn't take men's goods, he takes their lives and sells them. I'm leaving Kit."

Kit was silent.

"I mean I'm leaving."

"Where to?"

"Venice, there's a galley going to Venice for supplies. Kit, you're a brave one Kit."

"Shan't I see you again Deuce?"

"You won't even hear me. Kit …" He paused as if wondering whether to say it or not, "I know what you are, Kit, but I'll never tell anyone."

Deuce was gone. Kit wondered what he had meant.

Monday and the drums were beating. Once more the divisions were marching from the camp down to where the transports were moored waiting to carry them across the Golden Horn. Kit thought of the men who had marched down the hill from the castle of St. Foy and wondered if they were the same men as these silent, truculent, careworn creatures around him. There were certainly a lot less of them, perhaps half. They were a lot older, greyer and their eyes were not lifted with the promise of eternal life but set fixed with the almost certainty of death. There were one or two jokers amongst them, there will be jokers in hell but none in heaven. He missed having Thunderer at his side and smirked at Robert and Aimery stumbling on foot in their armour. The Squire had a boil on the back of his neck. Kit had never liked him.

The city could have been a range of mountains he was so used to the sight of it. The ships were in a long line and the divisions separated to board their allotted transports. He saw the Venetians had changed their tactics, each big transport had been lashed to another and the flying bridges now projected from the bows so that two attackers could fight side by side. Kit pointed it out to the Sergeant.

"You'll never get up there," said the Sergeant.

"Someone did."

"Yes and the poor fool fell off."

The Sergeant was not usually talkative but he went on.

"We're fighting next to the Venicers this time. It's the old Doge's idea. They're going right up to the walls and we're going where there's a bit of land by that gate." He pointed to the gate where Kit and Alaric had entered the city.

"It's blocked up," said Kit.

"Yes, it's blocked up."

"With bricks."

"With bricks," said the Sergeant. "You're a clever lad, you'll go far, if you ever get there."

Sergeants were well-known for their wit.

The transports were loaded and the ramps were hauled up. Kit was up on the forecastle with Robert's shield and sword propped up on the coil of rope on which he was sitting. Robert was talking to Aimery.

"If something should happen, no listen, leave me here. Go home Aimery, one of us must go home."

"God will look after you."

"We've let God down."

It was a new thought for Kit, that God could do nothing without man.

They were moving slowly across the water towards the end of the crusade. Whatever happened, victory or defeat, they would go no further than Constantinople. God would not save them.

"How far is it from the shore to the wall?"

Aimery did not know.

"I haven't been there."

"I have my lord." Kit spoke up and they turned to look at him.

"You?"

"I went with … I went to look."

"Against my orders? Of course it was. How far?"

"Within bow-shot."

"What's on the other side of the gate?"

"It's all burned down."

"Is there room to mount a charge?"

"Yes my lord, there's miles of it, it's huge!"

Aimery laughed. "Next time Robert, send a boy."

"We must break through the gate."

"It's brick, my lord."

"I know it's brick."

Aimery intervened. "He means it isn't stone. You can pull brick down, that's right isn't it Kit?"

"Yes my lord. You break a hole and …"

Robert cut him short. "We'll send the 'cats' in first."

Kit thanked Bishop in his head.

There were thousands of defenders on the towers and parapets and as the ships approached the shore they sent up a cheer and waved derisively as if to welcome them. Black smoke showed where the vats of oil and tar were being heated and some excited Greeks were loosing boulders from the engines on the towers that fell harmlessly but were a warning as the landing grew nearer.

Kit ran to the rail to see the Venetians heading straight at the wall with men in armour already on the bridges. His own turn came as he felt the ship grounding and ran down to wait amongst the men for the ramp to be lowered. On a grey morning, along a half-mile stretch of shore, Constantinople, the greatest city in the world, was being attacked by a puny force of desperate men.

Robert sent out his bowmen to try and deter the Greeks but they came under fiercer fire and the whirr of arrows carried the cries of men like seabirds. The sappers wheeled the "cats" ashore and ducked inside them where they were safe until they reached the wall and came under an avalanche of rocks. On the ramp Robert took his sword and shield but left his helmet with the Squire. He looked at Kit.

"Where's the hauberk I gave you?"

"My lord, I kept falling over in it, so I took it off."

"Stay close to me."

The company ran down the ramp and formed a line and immediately came within shot. Kit wished he had kept the hauberk. They advanced and the music of war, trumpets and drums, the Greek timbrels and gongs, the shouts and cries, the groans, the screams, struck up. Within bow-shot, three hundred yards to walk without showing any fear but fearfully, was the nearest Kit had got to hell so far. They halted under the wall and shouted warnings of falling rocks and missiles, whilst the "cats" were pushed up against the gate for the sappers to hack out the bricks with their pickaxes. Robert left with the Squire and Kit under his shield to direct the other companies of his division. They returned to the ship and climbed to the forecastle to oversee the assault as a whole.

Looking to the right towards the Blachernae palace where there was open ground, Montferrat's division was acting as a rearguard against any counterattack from the city. Flanders held the ground between them and Robert's division of Blois, while St. Pol was fighting from the Venetian transports and their flying bridges. It was St. Pol that made a vital breakthrough.

Two of the tallest ships, lashed together, were carried by the current and struck against a tower with a wooden superstructure bearing eight or nine Varangian Guards. A Venetian sailor on one of the bridges managed to scramble onto the tower where he was mercilessly cut down. This gave the chance for a knight in armour to cross from the second bridge, landing on his knees. Watching from the forecastle Robert cried out, "It's de Turboise I know his shield!" The Guards rushed at him and struck him several times and they heard the clang of axe on helmet. Kit thought that was the end of de Turboise, but no, the knight got to his feet and drew his sword. It was so far away it was like a puppet show and like a puppet show illogical. The Guards fell back. Perhaps they had had too many emperors to face an armed crusader and fight for another? A second knight leapt on to the tower, the Guards fled down a ladder, more soldiers and Venetians came across and the tower was taken. A man from St. Foy ran up to the ship and shouted, "My lord! The gate! We're through the gate!"

They hurried back, but at the gate there was the worst tragedy that Kit had seen. Greek fire had poured down onto the "cats" and set three of them alight. The flames could not be put out and the burning tar stuck to the hides which had dried up. Kit could only watch. The wooden roofs caved in and the men beneath them burned to death. It was as if he was alone and the only witness.

It took a moment for anyone to move. When they could they dragged the smoking blackened wood away. Nobody dared to touch the charred corpses underneath.

"Look!" Kit pointed.

There was a jagged opening in the brickwork.

Some of the soldiers took a step forward but immediately drew back for fear of treading on the dead. Whilst the action screamed and clashed around them, the group at the gate were silent spectators staring at the charred smouldering bodies piled up in an obscene and ghastly agglomeration. It would be sacrilege to climb over them. Kit hid behind Robert and Aimery fearing to look but looking and he saw the first man to move. A fat man pushed through, seized a pike from a soldier and trod from corpse to corpse as if he was on a country walk. Once at the gate he thrust the pike into the opening and began vigorously dislodging bricks. Others followed, picking a more respectful way across the dead and venting their rage and revulsion on the wall. Soon there was a gap low but wide enough for a man.

Aimery started forward but Robert restrained him. There was still the danger from above. Rocks were falling between them and the gate. In that moment the fat man pushed the others aside and forced his gross bulk between the bricks. He had to bend down and the last Kit saw of Bishop was the broad seat of his leather breeches.

They waited for the shout or cry that would announce his fate but none came. A soldier peered through the opening and drew back in alarm.

"There's thousands of them! Thousands!"

Aimery broke away from Robert, put on his helmet and unsheathed his sword. The men made way for him, dragging some of the corpses aside and he stooped to enter the gap. Robert tried to stop him, grabbing his foot, but he pulled himself through and disappeared. They heard the groan of an audience of thousands at some grand spectacle.

Aimery called out.

"My lord, come through! They're drawing back! They're beginning to run away!"

Had one man, as bold and brave as Aimery was, dispelled a crowd of thousands, or was he just the catalyst of their indifference and dismay? They had come to see the foreigners destroyed, they were disappointed, but the Emperor would pay not them. The citizens of Constantinople gave away the key of the door believing they would still keep the house when the burglars had gone.

Robert came through with the Sergeant and about forty men in armour from several companies. They stood and stared at the vast crowd which was slowly ebbing away, leaving the blackened ground and stark standing timbers like some deserted beach. Kit had come through the gate and looked up for any danger, but the defenders had gone from the walls all along the Golden Horn from the Blachernae palace to the sea. The impenetrable walls of Constantinople had been abandoned, the gates forced open and the city defeated by its own citizens.

Then, as if in defiance, they heard drums and timbrels banging and clanging, announcing that the Greek army was about to return and destroy them. They lined up with their backs to the wall. Robert ordered Kit to fetch Thunderer, if he was going to die it would be on horseback.

Kit left reluctantly and ran back through the gate to the shore where the transports had landed. Horses were coming off the ramps with the grooms boasting to each other of their bravery. He saw Alaric and was afraid of being rebuffed and ran up the ramp into the hold. The farrier had armed Aimery's horse but had not touched Thunderer. From the way he hobbled Kit guessed Thunderer had touched him. The farrier was a man of few foul words, "He's a bugger!" Thunderer was bucking and trampling. Kit dodged his hooves as he prepared him for battle.

Kit rode Thunderer down the ramp and along the shore to the gate. There were crusaders and Venetians everywhere. Robert's Squire was with the company outside the gate and he waved Kit through. He brought Thunderer to a shuddering halt! What he saw frightened him more than anything he had seen before.

Robert, Aimery, the Sergeant and a few men in armour, thirty or forty, were backed against the wall. Across the wasteland stood the best of the Greek army. They had not fought and could have been on parade in full-dress uniform with shining weapons, Guards, Greek soldiers and mercenaries. Standing out in front of them on a golden-caparisoned charger was the

Emperor, Mourtzouphlus, as splendid as his name in his gold helmet and grasping a silver mace. Kit turned to see a line of battle-weary men, haggard and unshaven, tired and tattered as the crosses on their shoulders and two lords wearing their honours on their heads and shields for perhaps the last time. There was no retreat and no defence.

Kit slid off Thunderer and led him to Lord Robert and helped him to mount. He stood by his lord's side. They were all as still as if they were at a funeral.

Mourtzouphlus raised the mace above his head and spurred the charger on. He rode a few paces and turned. Not one man in his army moved. He shouted a command, rode on a step or two and turned. No-one moved. He screamed in desperation and rode backwards and forwards along the line.

Kit glanced at Robert, as still as a statue and the men as still as spectators at a Roman circus of death.

Mourtzouphlus was bellowing insults at his army. Kit guessed they were insults because the Guards, the famous Varangians, turned their backs on the Emperor they were sworn to defend and marched away.

This was the signal for a mass defection and the Greeks, who had never fought, deserted their Emperor, not out of cowardice but disgust.

Mourtzouphlus turned to face his enemy. Kit feared some act of fatalism was about to take place.

This was not Rome but Constantinople, more civilised, more self-centred, more mercenary, more sensible. Mourtzouphlus trotted his horse a few paces towards them, made an obscene gesture and turned away, quickening to a gallop in case they chased him.

It struck Kit that this was no victory, no triumph, no glory, no crusade! It was the end of an empire, wretched, sad and unheroic. What had begun in St. Foy as the restoration of Christ's kingdom had ended here in the destruction of Christ's empire.

The sun declined and the Generals met to survey the situation. They were inside the city but only in the area flattened by the fire. They had not defeated the army or the people. Any advance would have to be into the narrow streets and between the houses and high buildings where they could be separated and trapped. No more could be done that night except to keep control of the troops. Orders were passed to the sergeants to command the men not to venture into the city and to lie on their arms all night.

Some were more comfortable than others. Kit heard that Count Baldwin had captured the Emperor's pavilion and slept in his bed while his men made do with the ground, forbidden to take even a carpet or a rug in case it was valuable.

This was the first instance of aristocratic stupidity and greed that principally contributed to the terror that was to come. Some of Baldwin's men went on the rampage, plundering the stores and warehouses and starting fires which spread to the dockyards along the Golden Horn. A great part of the trade of the city was destroyed. Kit saw the glow in the sky but did not know of the tragic folly that took place by its light until later. Some of the young pages from St. Pol decided to join in the fun and rode towards the fire. Greek girls and women were fleeing from their houses and a page on a fine horse was chasing a girl when his horse fell in a pit and Alaric broke his neck. It was a joke amongst the grooms and pages.

Mourtzouphlus had ridden back to the Great Palace cursing the disloyalty of his army. He rode into the streets seeking to arouse his people against the invaders. He might have been trying to arouse the stone emperors or the saints in their sepulchres or Saint Sophia herself. The people did not care who sat on the golden throne any more than who sat on a wooden one. The city was used to emperors in bloody comings and goings. The invaders had already put Alexius in the Great Palace and now had another candidate who would pay them to go away. Mourtzouphlus rode back, collected as many moveable treasures as he could, including old Isaac's widow and her three daughters who were said to be his mistresses and escaped in a fishing boat. Many of the great nobles, magnates and sycophants who had misruled the city from behind the throne now left for their country houses and estates. Others gathered in St. Sophia to elect a new emperor from their own ranks, a young man called Lascaris. They brought Lascaris before the Varangian Guard, the last authority in the city and asked for an oath of loyalty. The Varangians asked for an increase in their pay. Lascaris knew their oaths were now worthless and slipped away to take a passage in a galley going anywhere.

This was the preamble to the events of the next day that was just dawning, the 13th April 1204.

Kit had been awake most of the night and when dawn outlined the wall above his head he slipped out through the gate to look for water and feed for Thunderer. The ground was strewn with rocks and lumps of death. He went to the transport and found a bucket and a sack of straw. To fetch water he had to go back to the city. He knew from his outing with Alaric that the devastation caused by the fire stretched for a mile and set off for a domed building on higher ground. It was the monastery of Christ Pantepopos, Christ Who Sees Everything. The monks were at prayer. A dirty-looking boy with a bucket was not a surprise and a monk took Kit to the well. Kit wondered at their forbearance. Their city had been burnt and broken into, hated crusaders were within call. Whilst he was drawing water the monk even spoke to him in his own language.

"Who is to be the new emperor, the Marquis of Montferrat, no?"

Kit was amazed the monk could speak and knew more than he did.

"It doesn't matter, my son. Christ is our emperor."

Kit thought, no he isn't, Christ is a poor man, a common man.

"He rules the world."

He hung on a cross that's why I'm here.

"It does not matter which man is called emperor."

If it doesn't matter why did so many have to die?

"Christ gives you His blessings, my son."

Our priests call these priests Jews and dogs, the enemies of Christ and this priest blesses me in the name of Christ. Are there two Christs, or just two priests?

He carried the bucket down the hill. A bucket is a bucket.

The company was rising from the ground as the dead are supposed to do one day. Robert had taken Thunderer to ride to a council meeting in Montferrat's pavilion. Kit walked up the hill again.

The Generals had slept well. They had heard of Mourtzouphlus' defection and Lascaris' disappearance but the Varangian Guard and the Greek army were still intact. They expected to have to fight their way into the city street by street. There was no thought of negotiating a new treaty to enable the crusade to sail for the Holy Land. This was their Holy Land. Who was to be god?

Kit was outside the pavilion and was the first to see a procession coming from the centre of the city on foot. It was led by the Patriarch in his golden cope and tiara, accompanied by acolytes with icons and crosses. Officers of the Varangian Guard followed in their court uniforms and a string of merchants and shippers of all nations except Greek.

Kit ran in and told Robert who warned the Generals and they quickly agreed to refuse any terms they might be offered. They ranged themselves in seniority with Montferrat in the centre in suitably martial attitudes. The leaders of the deputation were allowed to enter and, to the Generals' surprise, prostrated themselves in front of Montferrat. He was the chosen one. They opened the city to him believing he had the supreme power over the crusader army and was therefore bound to be their next emperor. Montferrat was magnanimous, but Baldwin of Flanders, Hugh of St. Pol, Louis of Blois, were silent fuming pillars of mistrust and jealousy. The deputation backed away to prepare the city to welcome their new emperor. Montferrat turned to the Generals with a disarming smile and open hands, of course he could not be the new emperor yet. In that moment, the authority over the crusaders was dissipated by spite and not one of them acted to control his men and protect Constantinople from devastation.

Kit was standing outside the pavilion with the other grooms and pages when he heard angry voices and was astonished to see Montferrat and Baldwin jostling to get out and running to mount their horses and shouting orders to alert their companies and bring them into the city. They galloped off, Montferrat towards the Great Palace and Baldwin towards the Blachernae palace. The divisions and disasters started at the top. Hugh of St. Pol and Louis of Blois were more restrained but were equally anxious to go and claim the biggest house they could get. Robert appeared more modestly and shook his head.

"They rule whole countries. They're only men like us."

He got up on Thunderer. His ideals of honour, nobility, faith, all fallen with his idols.

"My lord, where are you going?"

"Kit?" It was as if Robert had woken from a dream. "To get myself a house, I suppose." The reality of broken faith is desperately sad.

Robert rode away. Kit thought he had better tell the Sergeant.

The Sergeant already knew. The army had split apart into three thousand atoms of uncontrollable lust and greed. He had managed to hold the men of St. Foy together and when Kit arrived breathless he made him sit under the wall they had won.

"You can't blame them. By law, if you besiege a city, you've got three days to take what you like, but it's more than that. They've broken every promise they've made to us since we set out and they've made us break our oaths to God. We've been away two years and where are we? Not in Jerusalem that's sure. How many dead son? You put up with it all like the rest of us. You know what the orders were? Any gold or silver or cloth you get worth more than five sous has got to go to the Provost Marshal to be divided up later. Like they did in Zara, divided it in two and took both."

"You won't take us to Lord Robert?"

"Who said that? He's the only good one there is. He'll look after us. Come on, lads. Listen, no women and no priests, alright?"

Kit did not know what he meant.

The men of St. Foy marched in fairly good order on the route taken by Kit and Alaric when they had visited the city for the first time. They halted at the church of the Apostles. It appeared to be deserted, the doors were wide open and Kit ran inside. At first he thought nothing had changed but, as his eyes darkened, he saw the altar had been stripped of its candlesticks and vessels. The door to the mausoleum of the emperors was sagging from one silver hinge, the other had been hacked out. He went in slowly. The floor was strewn with what looked like ashes and broken shards of pottery mixed with torn shreds of old cloth. The tombs appeared to be intact until he saw a slab of marble cracked across by a sapper's sledge-hammer and realised they had all been breached and robbed and the rubbish on the floor was the last resting-place of emperors. What diadems and golden torques and crucifixes now adorned crusaders? He ran away.

They marched through the poor quarter of the city where frightened slaves and servants peered from doorways wondering if they had to go to work, on to the Greek houses of thousands of clerks and artisans, shipwrights and sawyers, builders and blacksmiths, shopkeepers, empty corpuscles of a dying heart and on to the street and colonnade where the destructive plague was rampant. The army of God was going about its business.

Men were breaking into shops that sold things they had never seen before and stealing things they would never need, the delicacies and delights of a rich and decadent society. Kit saw a man with a Chinese wash-bowl clutched to his chest and another with a woman's hat. There was a mule they had found, loaded with furniture. The gold and silver had gone to the first wave of looters, but the second kept on stealing. The Sergeant marched them on, several with an envious glance aside.

The triumphal way, here - O God - was where the leading citizens, the officers of state, the lawyers, senators, the high members of the clergy, all with great ceremony and with their wives and children around them, had gathered to welcome the new Emperor, to pledge their loyalty and hopefully keep their jobs. Here, when the first crusaders appeared with weapons in their hands, they must have thought them barbarians without propriety, but perhaps normal in provincial Rome. A soldier wearing the cross put out a filthy hand to tear the necklace from a lady's neck, her husband moved to stop him and was struck down and stabbed to death. They were shocked by the flagrancy as much as the deed. It had never happened in Constantinople. Emperor had murdered emperor, politician politician, rival rival, but this blatant pointless slaughter outraged their culture as well as their humanity. They had no time to think or run. Blood begets blood and the soldiery were on them, robbing, killing and when the blood was up, violating women and girls as they lay in the public street by daylight, witnessed by the children.

Kit saw it all.

Robert had commandeered a large house facing the square of Constantine. He posted men to guard it against the crusaders. Kit found a refuge with Thunderer in the stables. He hid. What shreds of faith he had were shrivelled by cold terror and consumed by burning anger. Where was Christ? Not in this world. Poet's words came back to him, "You're the only one who thinks it's going to happen in this world, in this time, in this way." He would never get to Jerusalem, he would never fight for Christ, he would be like all the others.

It was a trick. The crusade had been honeycombed with falsehood, sweet and empty. As the blood in the chapel was false, so were the lies of the priest, the promises that were never meant to be kept. He brooded in the dark corner of the stable and began to hate himself for being tricked into going on crusade, his stupid childish belief he could help Christ. Christ did not help himself. Kit felt guilty, the dupe is guilty of being duped. He felt defiled by being. That was why Poet had gone to death, the shame and disgust of being. He glanced at Thunderer sleeping. Man is the only creature which rapes and murders. God's child the killer.

Well, if he was not a hero like Poet he could be a villain like Bishop. Bishop was not ashamed of anything and treated God like a brother, just as he treated Uncle Flyn, the king of tricks. Having decided he slept.

On the second day he went out with Lord Robert and the Squire thieving. Robert could see St. Sophia from his bedroom window so he decided to rob it first. He was too late. Busy unshaven men with dirty crosses on their shoulders were hacking at the great altar and huge mosaics to prise out a few precious fragments of jewel or gold. Others were ripping down hangings and drapery for the gold thread in them. All the precious treasures had gone to the first looters and these were breaking up furniture and fittings to load onto the stolen donkeys fouling the marble floor.

Robert led the way to the Great Palace where he was stopped by Montferrat's guards. The innumerable treasures collected by the emperors over the centuries were now the property of the Marquis. The Doge, who had moved in next door, had appropriated other securities for his old age, the crown of thorns, the robe of the Virgin, pieces of the True Cross, the head of John the Baptist, which he hoped would ensure his place in heaven.

There was a monastery nearby and a weeping monk bemoaned the loss of its greatest treasure, another head of John the Baptist. Kit began to wonder at the miracle.

A church produced a crystal cross for Robert and the Squire squeezed a small gold cross out of a priest.

Robert complained and hurried to the vast church requisitioned by the Provost Marshal to store all the gold, silver and cloth valued at more than five sous, to be fairly divided amongst the crusaders. The Provost Marshal was not there and the church echoed emptily with his laughter.

In every palace, church, monastery, mansion, house and hovel, the greatest robbery in the world had taken place. Constantinople was more desolate than Jerusalem after the Babylonians had been there.

Where were the people? Thousands had fled to the west, risking pillage, rape and death at the hands of rapacious bands of crusaders. They had walked the way, not of triumph but humiliation, defeated by their own complacency and belief.

Robert returned with the single hope he might secure a fiefdom in the coming carve-up of the empire.

On the third day Kit woke up wondering what was going to happen to him. The crusade was over. The Venetians would take their money and ship their stolen treasures to Venice. Old Dandolo would stay in his sequestered palace to oversee the depredation of his half of the city. Lord Robert would follow Count Louis on the trail of murder and extortion. He would not lie in a crusader's tomb. Kit could neither go nor stay. He lay on his straw bed and thought more than he had ever thought before and thought of nothing. It is impossible to think of nothing for long. A door slammed somewhere, Thunderer turned his head, the straw mattress was suddenly like a bed of torture. He sat up and grasped his last hope - Bishop. What would Bishop do? Bishop would survive. He must have done, there was no Bishop on the other side of the wall. Bishop would steal enough to pay a ship's master to take him to a friendly harbour, buy a donkey and go home. Kit laughed at himself, Bishop would do more than that but it would do for Kit! He jumped up and put on his working clothes but kept his cross, there would be crusaders in the streets. This was all the cross meant to him now. He stroked Thunderer for luck, he would be back but with his future in his pocket.

It was still early but there were gangs of crusading vultures around. The huge corpse of Constantinople would last them sixty years. He knew where he was going. Alaric had taken him there twice and Bishop had been in the kitchen. It was well away from the great public squares and buildings, the shops and stores, it was deliberately unfashionable and he knew how to get in. Beyond the empty grandeur of domes and columns, mocked by drunken shouts of once decent men and caws of well-fed crows and ravens, the streets narrowed and the houses were drab, tall and shuttered. There was nothing gaudy here for the predators. There were stray groups of three or four grey-faced crusaders with blue and yellow crosses as if they were the stigmata of some deadly disease, some in stolen garments, others grasping worthless trifles, who barely glanced at the boy with the red cross as if he was uneatable. It was quiet and clear in the street he wanted, some drifts of sea-rack in the sky, the houses looked deserted. He came to the steps he had sat on and, with a quick look around, slipped out of sight into the area. He squeezed through the window into the cellar and cautiously climbed the steps. There was no one in the corridor or the kitchen. They all must have fled at the first alarm. Had they taken the money with them? He looked in all the alcoves, there were glasses on the tables, they must have left in a hurry. He climbed the staircase to a landing. The carpet was thicker and there were several rooms. Some of the doors were open and he saw stuffed chairs and thick covers, beds and mirrors, but there were no chests under the beds or caskets on the gilt tables and he began to think he was in the wrong place.

There was another, narrower staircase but he had already decided to leave. What made him look once more? The mirror. Kit had never seen himself in a mirror. Fatal mirror!

It was a full-length mirror and in it he saw a short fat boy with a round freckled face and mousy hair, wearing dirty stable-clothes and a once-white ribbon with a faded red cross. He pulled a face at himself, disappointed he was not the brave steel-clad knight who had set out for Jerusalem to fight for Christ. He tugged the ribbon and dropped it on the floor. It meant nothing to him now.

He was fascinated by the room. Pale yellow April morning sunlight softened the garish reds and golds, the stains of old encounters, the gilt and guilt of the past. Kit thought it the sort of room he would have liked in St. Foy. He sat in a chair and plumped up and down. He got up to look at a dressing-table with a blonde wig on a stand and pretty little bottles and pots of scent, creams and red powder. He was tempted to put his finger in a pot and put a spot of red powder on his nose. He looked in the mirror and rubbed it off. There was a wardrobe figured with a frieze of Greek women in gauzy garments and he opened it to see a line of multicoloured dresses and chemises and shoes with silver buckles. He went back to sit in the chair. In the warmth of the morning the richness of the room and aroma of cheap scent and old sweat enveloped him. He wanted to touch the dresses and went to the wardrobe and felt the silks and there was a collar of vair or ermine he pulled out and put around his neck. He looked in the mirror and grimaced at himself as a boy would and then adjusted it to fit. He sat in the chair. He went to the door to look out onto the landing and to listen and came back and sat in the chair. He was drawn to the wardrobe and chose a dress, not the first or second but carefully. He took a yellow dress and went to the mirror to hold it against himself. He laughed and put it back. He sat down and rose immediately and chose a red dress and stroked the silk and held it against his face. His eyes were soft as if all the horrors he had seen since he left St. Foy had faded and he was in another dream. He went to put the dress back and suddenly turned and laid it on a chair. O God, poor Kit!

He took off his jacket, pushed down the breeches and stepped out of them. He was in the dirty undervest he had never taken off. He could not put the beautiful dress over that and he pulled it over his head and dropped it as if he was sloughing a skin. He held the red dress up and down, deeply engaged in how to put it on. It was too full to go over his head and eventually he laid it on the floor, stepped into it and drew it up. He worked his arms into the tight sleeves and turned to look in the mirror. He saw a boy in a dress.

Kit was in the grip of a transformation he could neither understand nor stop. He took the wig from the dressing-table and put it on. Now he was a boy in a wig and a dress. He went back to the table and became absorbed in the creams and powders, moving between the table and the mirror, so absorbed he did not hear the sound. He primped and posed in the mirror, in fun and in earnest. He turned to the wardrobe for a pair of buckled shoes and saw the man in the doorway. He was surprised but not afraid, here was a crusader filthy unshaven holding a short sword. He had seen thousands of them and lived amongst them and was one himself. The man's eyes slitted, he raised his head and drew his lips tight to show his teeth. Kit had seen a wolf do it. He screamed! God, he was a boy, why did he scream? Because he was no longer a boy.

The man shouted something and five or six more came up to see what he had found. It took no time. Kit fought but the first man turned the sword round and struck him with the hilt, splitting the skull from temple to cheek. The blessed oblivion of death spared Kit from what followed.

~

Part Four

~

KIT DIED but Kitty lived. She lay in the bed for days, perhaps weeks, tended by the women who had been hiding in the attic. They helped her out of pity and the thought that she had suffered the horrors meant for them. Her wounds were fearful, her face scarred, blinded in one eye, her body ravaged and torn. Only the elemental power of nature had kept her alive, or God. God in return for the oath she had taken in the chapel at St. Foy to give her life to Christ.

Outside in the city many of the crusaders had gone on campaign with Baldwin, who had been made emperor to spite Montferrat and was now attempting to conquer his empire. Others had joined Montferrat, angry and thwarted, on a futile adventure in Thessaly. Those who had stayed used their stolen gold and silver to make the brothel thrive. Lust knows no nationalities. The alcoves were occupied and the rooms were open, except for the one where Kitty lay in the room Kit would have liked. The madam had fled with her fortune and the women had bribed one of the Generals to give them the house.

Constantinople would survive, but had suffered as Kitty had suffered, rape and rapine. The crusader emperors took what they could move and destroyed what they could not, melting down Greek statues for coinage, stripping the fabric of the churches, selling the stones and marble, mortgaging the once great commerce for ready money. Relics worshipped for centuries appeared in abbeys and churches all over Europe, often the same in one city as another.

Those lords and officers, Robert, Aimery, the Sergeant, who could afford the passage sailed home with stories of great courage in taking a Christian city by storm,when it was lost by apathy.

When Kitty could rise she never left the house. Most of Kit's memories had been excised by the short sword. She could still see Thunderer and Bishop, she mercifully forgot Poet, but remembered the old Jew. She believed she was being punished for the death of the old Jew. A people was punished for the death of a young Jew. The women kept her and gave her a bucket to scrub the kitchen floor.

With the years the women changed but Kitty stayed and became a familiar figure, cleaning, cooking, caring for the new young girls. In time she was paid with gratuities, though she never saw the clients in case they saw her. She never wanted to see another man. Sometimes an old crusader would pay for his comfort with a stolen relic which the girls gave her. This was as near as Kitty ever got to Jerusalem.

She aged quickly. Constantinople aged, old Dandolo was buried in St. Sophia, a poor exchange for its past glories. Perhaps Jerusalem was fortunate these crusaders never got there, although Jerusalem was never fortunate for long. Kitty had been in the house for many years, I remember, when she had enough money to buy a passage in a sailing ship destined for Marseilles. She put her relics in a package and a veil over her face and left the house for the first time as Kitty. In Marseilles, as Kit had once promised, she bought a donkey and made the perilous journey to St. Foy. Nobody bothered the old woman and if a man approached her she raised her veil. She had no memory of St. Foy and went there only because she knew of nowhere else to go. As she entered the town and passed the road to the castle, she saw an old black horse cropping grass in a field. She smiled, she had seen him somewhere else before.

She rode her donkey to the priory and told the nun who answered the bell she had a gift for them. The relics were received with rapture, nobody knew who St. Foy might have been and St. Stephen's finger was a treasure beyond belief. In the chapel she saw a new-cut tomb with the effigy of a crusader which, she never told them, should not have covered Lord Robert. She was gladly accepted into the order of nuns and given a new name. In time she was elected prioress.

Yes, I was Kitty.

One day, how many years later I do not remember, a nun ran in to say there was a great cleric, a bishop and his train, who had stopped on the way to Lyons to ask if anyone knew what had happened to a boy called Kit from St. Foy. I said, "Tell his Grace, God bless him, no, nobody knows a word."